THE KILLER BAT

COVID 19: Origin & Ramifications

PANDEMIC 2020
Theory of Animal Viruses

G. ASHISH KALRA

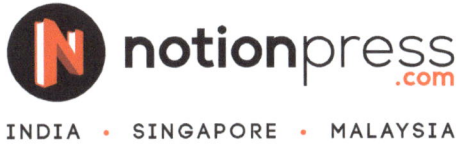

INDIA · SINGAPORE · MALAYSIA

Notion Press Media Pvt Ltd

No. 50, Chettiyar Agaram Main Road,
Vanagaram, Chennai, Tamil Nadu – 600 095

First Published by Notion Press 2021
Copyright © G. Ashish Kalra 2021
All Rights Reserved.

ISBN
Hardcase 978-1-68563-931-0
Paperback 978-1-68586-619-8

This book has been published with all efforts taken to make the material error-free after the consent of the author. However, the author and the publisher do not assume and hereby disclaim any liability to any party for any loss, damage, or disruption caused by errors or omissions, whether such errors or omissions result from negligence, accident, or any other cause.

While every effort has been made to avoid any mistake or omission, this publication is being sold on the condition and understanding that neither the author nor the publishers or printers would be liable in any manner to any person by reason of any mistake or omission in this publication or for any action taken or omitted to be taken or advice rendered or accepted on the basis of this work. For any defect in printing or binding the publishers will be liable only to replace the defective copy by another copy of this work then available.

This Book is dedicated to

a. *My Fantastic Mother*
b. *My Advisers and Gurus at the University of Texas at Austin (#1 University in the World)*

    - Dr. Sten Thore, Professor of Mathematical Economics, The University of Texas at Austin & Professor, IC2 Institute, The University of Texas at Austin

    - Dr. George Kozmetsky, President, IC2 Institute, The University of Texas at Austin & Founder, Graduate School of Business at the University of Texas at Austin

Vote of Thanks

I would personally like to thank some extraordinary people who went out of their way to provide valuable suggestions during this last 19 months since the Pandemic broken out in Wuhan. First, I would like to thank Jaitirth Rao, ex CEO of Citibank India for his valuable comments and advice at the start and making me believe that there was a "road ahead" for my work. Second, I would like to thank Mudit Jain, President of the DCW Group for his sincere and valuable advice over the last 15 months. Mudit is a staunch vegetarian and had highlighted some of the issues of being "non vegetarian" over ten years back. His thinking made me also delve deeper into the beautiful aspects of Jainism and its relevance in addressing some of the issues we have faced during this Pandemic. Ingrid Newkirk, Founder and Chief at PETA has been fabulous with her encouragement and kind words, which have been very highly appreciated. I have been hugely inspired by the tremendous and resilient efforts of PETA to structure a better and more equitable world for Humans & Animals.

I would also like to thank Ravindra Asundi and his younger brother Dr. Jai Asundi, both dear friends, for their advice and helping me navigate through some difficult problems. Jai's advice around some Vegan diets and helping me think through the title of the book has been extremely value added. I am indebted to all the above for their advice, patience and sharing their knowledge and lessons from their valuable experience with me.

Bats' role in the Animal Ecosystem

The Bat plays a key role in the Animal Ecosystem. They pollinate over 500 flowers, and eat mosquitoes that are harmful to Human Beings. Bats inject Bat Coronaviruses in various Animals. Bat Coronaviruses get transferred to various Animals (Horses, Pigs, Camels, Civets, Pangolin, Ferret Badgers) and even domestically reared Animals (Cattle, Pigs and Chicken). Furin Cleavage sites are present in all Bat Coronaviruses. These Bat Coronaviruses get transferred to Human Beings when we eat these Animals via the Furin Cleavage Sites. Human consumption of Animals has caused Deadly Viruses in the past 75-100 years that have included the Asian Flu Pandemic (Human Consumption of Ducks, 1958-59), Swine Flu Pandemic (Pigs, 2009), The Deadly SARS Virus (Civets, 2002-2003), MERS Virus (Camels, 2012) and now COVID 19 (Pangolin/Ferret Badgers, 2020). In this process, Bats "protect the Animal Ecosystem" from encroachment by the Human Ecosystem. These Deadly Viruses and Pandemics are deadly for Human Beings.

"Treat the earth well
It was not given to you by your parents
It was loaned to you by your children
We do not inherit the earth from our ancestors
We borrow it from our children"

– **Native American Proverb**

Contents

Introduction 11

Chapter 1   History of Animal Viruses 17

Chapter 2   COVID 19: Understanding Coronaviruses 29

Chapter 3   COVID 19: Why Can't I Eat Beef, Chicken
or Pork, Please? 39

Chapter 4   Wuhan & Why We Didn't Learn from SARS? 49

Chapter 5   Understanding [(A-H) + (H-H) Raise to N]
Transmission 57

Chapter 6   COVID 19: Why the Lab Theory is Bogus! 63

Chapter 7   Why Have Most of the Major Viruses
Come from China? 97

Chapter 8   "Bat Coronaviruses: The Role of the
Furin Cleavage Site" 105

Chapter 9   COVID 19: Why Variants Will Defeat Vaccines 111

Chapter 10 Eleven Madison Park Goes MEATLESS......................... 121

Chapter 11 Why We Need Each Other –
"A Nudge to Vegetarianism".. 131

Conclusion... 137

Introduction

The Title of this Book is "The Killer Bat: COVID 19: Origin and Ramifications". Bat Coronaviruses get transferred to various Animals (Horses, Pigs, Camels, Civets, Pangolin, Ferret Badgers) and even domestically reared Animals (Cattle, Pigs and Chicken). These Bat Coronaviruses get transferred to Human Beings when we eat these Animals. These have caused Deadly Viruses in the past 75-100 years that have included the Asian Flu Pandemic (1958-59), Swine Flu Pandemic (2009), The Deadly SARS Virus (2002-2003), MERS Virus (2012) and now COVID 19 (Pangolin/Ferret Badgers). In this process, Bats "protect the Animal Ecosystem" from encroachment by the Human Ecosystem. These Deadly Viruses and Pandemics are deadly for Human Beings. Thus, the title, "The Killer Bat".

Crows are Black. They are born black. In a very rare case, you see a White Crow. This Pandmeic is a very rare random Event. Mathematically, it is very rare. These events happen once in a million or sometimes once in 100 years like the current Pandemic. Sometimes these events are not pleasant, but happen for a reason. They are probabilistically necessary.

I started solving the problem of "The White Crow" in my senior year at the University of Texas at Austin at the IC2 Institute in 1993 where I was blessed to work with 2 of my Advisers (Gods), Dr. Sten Thore, Norwegian School of Economics who was a Mathematical Economist who worked for the President of the Institute, the Amazing Dr. George Kozmetsky. Both of them were the finest, most refined, intellectually gifted and kindest Human Beings I have ever met. Dr. Kozmetsky motivated me to continue working with this initial problem of Newton's Law and its applicability to social problems. One of the latter chapters addresses the problem. The hypotheses started with studying of the Marburg problem in 1964 in Germany, Superman (Christopher Reeves) in a wheelchair and lessons from the Asian Flu Pandemic (1959, China). Dr. Thore, to whom I am eternally grateful for teaching me the best class of my Life at the IC2 Institute wrote back to me on my 6 hypotheses, in a beautifully typed letter in the Fall of 1993 "Ashish this is very good, very good. Do not lose sight of it, Do not lose sight of it, Never lose sight of it". The genesis of the Pandemic is from my work at the IC2 Institute at the World's No 1 University, The University of Texas at Austin. This Equilibrium that will emerge will be called "The Kozmetsky Thore Equilibrium".

We are at the fag-end of 2021 and, even at this juncture, we are still threatened and hampered by a virus that entered our lives in 2019. COVID-19 has wreaked havoc on the lives and livelihoods of almost all the people on the globe, and it has reached epic pandemic proportions, disrupting human life and businesses on a global scale. There have been scores of deaths and hospitalisations which left people vulnerable to future health issues, along with tremendous loss of economic growth and unmitigated damage to quality of life and business. People have been relegated to their homes, tourism has come to a standstill and on-ground education has suffered woeful injuries in the course of the pandemic. The damage done to the healthcare sector and frontline workers is unprecedented.

As soon as the virus emerged as a threat to humankind, the global scientific and medical community came together and worked ceaselessly tirelessly to envisage the right medical response to the ongoing COVID-19 pandemic. While we have met with some success, and vaccination drives are underway in several countries, there is always a concern regarding the appearance of newer strains and the possibility of infection even after being double vaccinated. The larger question revolves around the probability of nipping the COVID virus, as well as other similar pathogens, in the bud and the key to this future possibility lies in first understanding these unique animal viruses, studying their origins, identifying key transmission routes, and then attempting to overcome the same in a sustainable and resilient manner.

Since its origin, humanity has always been threatened by different strains and families of animal viruses. What, then, is an animal virus? An infectious agent that is incapable of replicating outside a living animal cell is termed as an animal virus and the speciality of such viruses lies in the fact that they contain only one type of nucleic acid, either DNA or RNA. This peculiar characteristic makes them different from other intracellular obligatory parasites such as chlamydoae and rickettsiae bacteria. Most of the animal virus diseases affecting humans, especially the ones that are now confined to just humans and absent in animals, have their origins in humans' contact with domestic and wild animals and such infections have seen a rise over the past 11,000 years.

Studying the zoonotic diseases, or illnesses which jump from animals to human beings, have a startling common factor – new pathogens emerging from animals, especially viruses, have a high unpredictability factor and these continue to emerge and spread across the countries, leading to global pandemics similar to the one affecting the population currently, the novel coronavirus. Coronaviruses are a family of viruses that cause diseases in mammals and birds. In humans, seven different types have been identified, four of which are responsible for mild respiratory diseases while the other three cause more significant damage. The common cold originates from a mild version of a coronavirus while the SARS-CoV was responsible for 2002-2003 SARS which spread to 28 countries and claimed 774 lives by 2003. MERS-CoV broke out in Saudi Arabia in 2012 and was deadlier than SARS but less contagious – it killed 858 people. In 2019, SARS-Cov2 brought the COVID-19, which is considered more contagious than SARS, but has milder symptoms. However, since it is more widespread than any of the others, up to date the global death tally is over 4.5 million.

The entire family of coronaviruses is thought to originate from animals. The exact origination of patient zero is still unclear, however, there are several theories for the same and the investigation is ongoing.

The current consensus stands that SARS-Cov2 originated sometime between October to November 2019. The first confirmed case was identified in the Wuhan province in China. And then it spread across the globe via human transfer. The globe is becoming increasingly interconnected, with globalisation a major trend in recent years, and this offers viruses further scope to affect global populations and evolve into life-threatening pandemics. The absence of specific treatment options and frequent viral mutations have created additional panic among humankind.

Consistent research and study into the virus have resulted in a startling discovery – we are, in part, responsible for the origin of zoonotic diseases in humans, as well as its future mutations. It is becoming increasingly clear that certain diseases can actually germinate from the food we eat. It is a well-known fact that infectious organisms, including pathogenic protozoans, bacteria and viruses have the ability to mutate and infect another host, despite being adapted to a particular animal host in the beginning of its lifecycle. While there are several instances of infectious agents in animal hosts altering themselves to infect human beings, such cases have not been seen in plant viruses. With the innate capability to transform itself based on the host body, animal viruses find it extremely easy to move from animals to human beings, and one of the major ways this happens is through ingestion. In fact, the eating habits of human beings have caused a number of preventable epidemics as well as an array of ailments in different parts of the body. In addition, environmental sustainability is also enhanced by the consumption of plant-based food items.

Considering the inherent risk in certain food groups, beef, chicken, and pork are known to be the most dangerous. Recent outbreaks of the COVID-19 infection at abattoirs and meat cutting plants in Germany have caused panic among individuals. Reports state that the virus affected employees at livestock facilities more than any other sector. While the lack of social distancing given the high capacity of such plants is one reason, there is also a strong possibility that the virus affected people because of their close contact with the high-risk food groups such as beef, pork and chicken.

My hypothesis is that the Variant B1617 (India variant) is caused due to the human consumption of chicken. There is Animal-Human Transmission and then Human to Human Transmission, followed by an exponential rise in transmission and subsequent infection in human beings. Such viruses ultimately have a domino effect on the population and this has been witnessed in the case of several animal viruses in the past, including Nipah (1997), Ebola (Bats,1997 and 2013), Swine Flu Pandemic (2009) SARS (Civets, 2003), MERS (Camels, 2004) and now COVID 19. Considering this life-threatening possibility, and the fact that consistent mutation in viruses is leading to inefficacy in vaccines, it is imperative that we, as a species, re-evaluate our food habits and evolve into more sustainable and flexible beings, conscious of what we consume and how it affects not just ourselves but the population at large.

Chapter 1

History of Animal Viruses

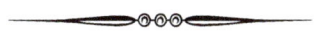

"Tell me what you eat, and I will tell you what you are."

– **Anthelme Brillat-Savarin**

ANIMAL VIRUSES are driven by the human consumption of animals over the last 100 years. These include but are not limited to Zika, Ebola, Asian Flu Pandemic, Swine Flu Pandemic, SARS, MERS, and the current COVID 19 Pandemic. The viruses have been most devastating, including the Asian Flu Pandemic, Swine Flu Pandemic, SARS, MERS, and the current COVID 19 Pandemic. More alarmingly, the intensity of the viruses has been increasing gradually as we move from viruses like Zika, Nipah (Human consumption of Bat infected Pigs) and SARS to the Swine Flu Pandemic(Pigs), MERS (Camels), and then to the COVID-19 Pandemic. Before we delve further into what animal viruses are and how they are threatening the human ecosystem, let us glance through some of the terrifying pandemics in history.

Exhibit 1: Increasing intensity of viruses

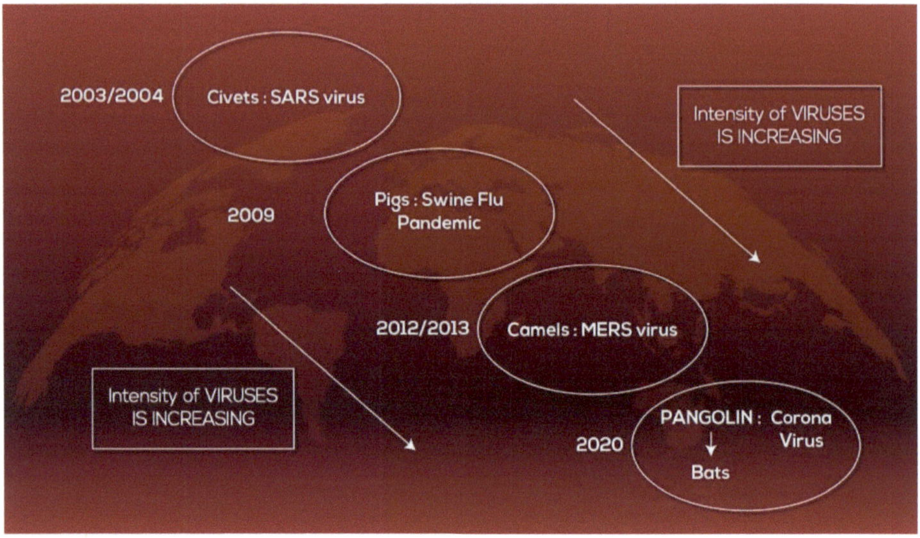

1.1 Major Pandemics in the History of Mankind

1. ASIAN FLU PANDEMIC (1958-59) (H2N2 VIRUS)

The Asian Flu Pandemic was a global Pandemic of Influenza A virus subtype H2N2 originated in Guizhou in Southern China. The number of deaths estimated due to this virus was between 1.5 million to 4 million people. This was mainly an Asian Pandemic. According to the CDC, there were 116,000 deaths in the United States. Also, the cause of this Pandemic was attributed to the human consumption of Ducks. According to Edwin Kilbourne, in "Influenza Pandemics of the 20th century," mentions that evidence suggests "those true pandemics with changes in hemagglutinin subtypes arise from genetic reassortment with Animal Influenza A viruses." Maurice Hilleman played a key role in identifying the beginning of a Flu Pandemic in 1957. According to the US Center for Disease Control & Prevention, the Asian Bird Flu was caused by the H2N2 virus, mutated from "wild ducks" and combined with a "pre-existing human strain." A vaccine was developed for it in 1958, and the deceleration of the Pandemic started, and it became part of the regular seasonal flow.

2. 1968 HONG KONG FLU PANDEMIC (1958-59) (H3N2 VIRUS)

The 1968 Pandemic was caused by Influenza A (H3N2 Virus) from a combination of 2 genes, an Avian Influenza A virus and the 1957 H2N2 virus. According to the Center for Disease Control & Prevention, there were around 1 million deaths worldwide and over 100,00 deaths in the United States. The H3N2 virus continues to circulate as a seasonal influenza A virus. Seasonal H3N2 viruses are typically associated with older people.

3. SWINE FLU PANDEMIC (2009)

The Swine Flu Pandemic was different from the H1N1 virus. Few young people had any immunity to this virus. This was also known as the (H1N1) pdm09 virus infection. The reason for the Swine Flu Pandemic was attributed to human consumption of "Pigs". CDC estimated that 151,700-575,000 people worldwide died from the H1N1 virus. At the peak, it was estimated that there were over 60.8 million cases and over 275,000 hospitalizations due to this Pandemic.

4. SARS Virus (2002, Civets, Guangdong, China)

The deadly SARS virus emerged in Guangdong, China. This is also known as the SARS-COV virus. The spread of the virus was very similar to what has happened with COVID 19. In "Science," June 2020, Robert Ross concludes, along with several Virologists, that the human consumption of Civets was the cause of the SARS virus. The mechanics of the spread of the virus is explained in Chapter 4. The SARS virus spread from a room in the Metropole in Hong Kong (from a nurse and Dr. Liu working on the SARS virus) to his fellow residents in the Hotel. They boarded planes to Singapore, Vietnam, Canada, Ireland, and the United States. Within 24 hours, the virus from Liu had spread to 5 Countries. SARS finally appeared in 32 Countries (Source: "Pandemic" by Sonia Shah, Harper Collins, 2020).

5. MERS Virus (2012, Camels, Middle East)

The deadly MERS virus emerged in the Middle East, mainly in Saudi Arabia. It was caused by human consumption of "Camels." MERS is a respiratory coronavirus by a novel Coronavirus (Middle East Respiratory Syndrome Virus). Over 37% of patients with MERS have died. According to a study by the World Health Organization, dromedary camels have been the major reservoir host for MERS-COV & an animal source of infection of MERS in humans. MERS has been one of the deadly diseases of this Century. The one big difference between MERS and COVID 19 is that the virus was localized in the case of MERS. In COVID 19, the virus spread because of regular flights after the Chinese New Year to Europe, United States, and Iran.

Exhibit 2: The mega viruses

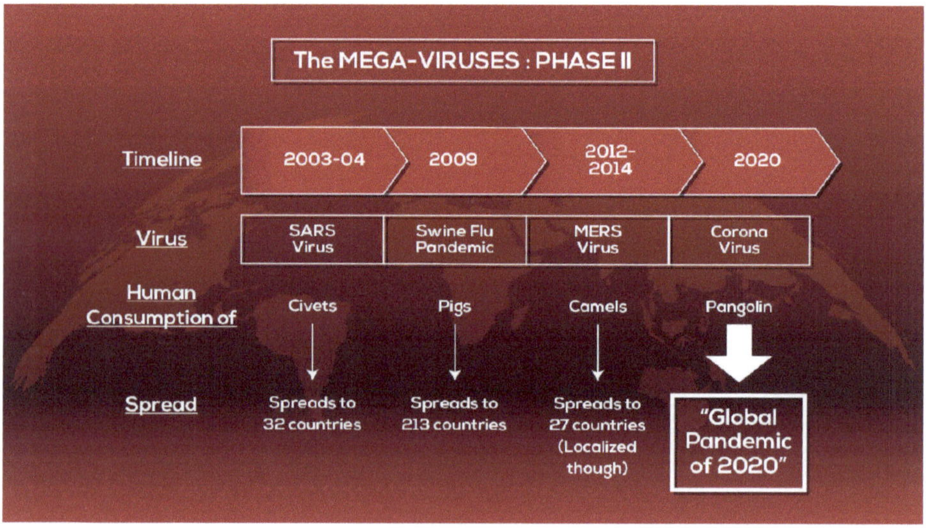

Timeline	2003-04	2009	2012-2014	2020
Virus	SARS Virus	Swine Flu Pandemic	MERS Virus	Corona Virus
Human Consumption of	Civets	Pigs	Camels	Pangolin
Spread	Spreads to 32 countries	Spreads to 213 countries	Spreads to 27 countries (Localized though)	"Global Pandemic of 2020"

1.2 What are Animal Viruses?

Animal viruses have always been a cause for concern when it comes to humankind. These viruses, which are typically immune to the action of antibiotics, are basically small infectious agents that are incapable of replicating outside a living animal cell. A speciality of such viruses is the fact that they contain only one type of nucleic acid, which could be either deoxyribonucleic acid (DNA) or ribonucleic acid (RNA). This makes them different from other intracellular obligatory parasites such as chlamydoae and rickettsiae bacteria.

Animal viruses do not replicate through the process of binary fission. Instead, they leverage the host cell's metabolism to replicate and they do this by diverting the cell's metabolism into synthesizing viral building blocks which are capable of self-assembling into new virus particles. These newly formed virus particles are then released into the body or the outer environment. The replication process requires cellular metabolic energy, various cellular enzymes, and cellular organelles. Interestingly, the viruses are incapable of producing this on their own. Therefore, they cannot survive outside a host cell.

While the animal virus is yet to attach itself to a living cell, it is termed as a virion and the terminology virus is only applied during the different phases of intracellular development. Virions are microscopic agents measuring between 20 to 300 nanometres in diameter and, given their minute size, they pass through filters that are capable of containing bacteria and other infectious bodies. However, there are some virions which may be 300 nm in diameter and they exceed the size of some of the comparatively smaller bacteria. Most virions are made up of proteins and nucleic acids but a few may also possess a lipid-filled membranous covering. The virions' protein molecules are organized in a symmetrical shell around the DNA or RNA, and these are termed as capsids. The shell and the nucleic acidtogether form the nucleocapsid.

Virions have exhibited two basic shapes and these are spherical and cylindrical. High resolution microscopes have revealed that the spherical viruses are polyhedral in morphology while the cylindrical virions possess helical symmetry. However, some virions do not depict any discernible features of symmetry and these virions are termed as complex virions. Classification is also made on the basis of virions containing DNA and RNA, as well as between virions with naked and enveloped nucleocapsids. It is the outer protein shell which protects the most important component of the virions – the viral genome. The shell protects the viral genome, which carries information specifying viral structure and functional components and enables the initiation and establishment of the infection cycle and generation of new virus, from destructive enzymes such as ribonucleases or deoxyribonucleases.

Most naked viral nucleic acids, when introduced into a susceptible cell by chemical or mechanical routes, lead to infections. The only exceptions to this rule are negative-strand RNA viruses and RNA tumour viruses. Animal viruses are more dangerous than bacteria as they cannot be treated with antibiotics. A viral infection consists of several steps including adsorption, penetration, uncoating and eclipse, and maturation and release and these spread through channels such as dust, aerosols, direct contact with carriers, and by bites or stings from animal and insect vectors which house the virus. The first stage of infection, or adsorption, occurs on specific receptors present in the membrane of an animal cell. The cell's susceptibility of viral infections is decided by the presence or absence of such receptors. Viruses which possess envelope shells usually have surface spikes which are involved in adsorption but most animal viruses do not exhibit such enabling structures.

The next stage is penetration, which involves the invagination and ingestion of the virion by the cell membrane. Then comes the uncoating of the nucleic acid or the nucleocapsid, depending on the composition of the virus. This stage marks the disappearance of the original virion and ensures that viral infectivity cannot be recovered from the diseased cells. The next stage of the infection process is eclipse and, in this stage, the biochemical functions of the animal cell are manipulated to synthesize viral proteins and nucleic acids. Following eclipse, the last stage of the infection and replication comes into play. During the maturation and release phase, the virus's protein shell is assembled and the nucleic acid is inserted into it, following which the virus is released into other cells or the environment, leading to further infection.

1.3 Origins of Major Infectious Diseases

Humankind has suffered from and combated a number of infectious diseases since evolution. Most of these diseases, especially the ones that are now confined to just humans and absent in animals, have their origins from humans' contact with domestic and wild animals. ANIMAL VIRUSES driven by the human consumption of animals have emerged for the last 100 years. (Mad Cow Disease: Human consumption of CATTLE), (H5N1: CHICKEN), (Avian Flu in China, 1959: caused due to Human Consumption of Ducks), Nipah Virus was caused due to Human Consumption of Pigs (Source: CDC). The deadly Swine Flu Pandemic, 2009, was also because of Pigs. Human consumption of Bats in West Africa caused the Ebola Virus (Source: COVID 19 by Deborah MacKenzie).

Exhibit 3: Animal viruses caused due to proximity to and human consumption of, animals

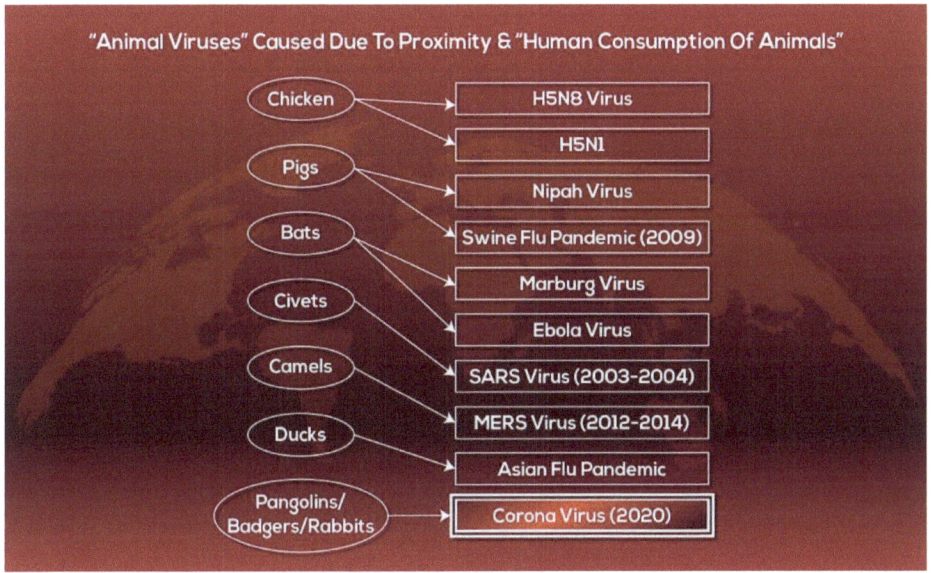

There are five intermediate stages of transition which lead a pathogen, which exclusively affects animals, to evolve into a pathogen which exclusively targets human cells. The diseases originated from humans' hunter/gatherer phase, wherein they were in constant contact with wild primates, creating an environment conducive to transfer of infectious pathogens and viruses. However, the infectious diseases that followed this stage were prompted by agriculture, for humans began to form colonies and settle in groups, making the whole community susceptible to an infection caught by one individual. Such infections have seen a rise over the past 11,000 years and did not exist before the origin of agriculture because, before agriculture, humans did not live in colonies.

The spread of infectious diseases has also had a major impact on world history – in fact, it is suggested that Europeans were unable to conquer Old World Tropical lands because of the prevalence of diseases which infected them and forced them to retreat or perish. This was also the reason behind French Emperor Napoleon Bonaparte's inability to conquer Russia. The phenomenon which leads to a human getting infected from an animal vector is termed zoonoses. Diseases and infections which are naturally transmitted between vertebrate animals and humans are included under zoonoses and these can be further classified under three segments – endemic zoonoses, epidemic zoonoses and emerging and re-emerging zoonoses.

Endemic zoonoses are found in many geographical locations and affect a large number of people and animals, while epidemic zoonoses are sporadic in spatial and temporal distribution. The third category of zoonoses, which includes yellow fever, SARS, H1N1 2009 and Avian flu, among others, are infections which are either newly appearing in a population or have been in existence previously but are now increasing rapidly in incidence and geographical range. Reports estimate that, globally, zoonoses cause about one billion cases of illness and millions of deaths on a yearly basis and, about 60% of globally emerging infectious diseases are classified as zoonoses, depicting the huge quantum of diseases which are transferred from animals to humans.

1.3 The Origins and Impact of Recent Viruses

The new zoonotic diseases affecting humankind have a startling common factor – new pathogens emerging from animals, especially viruses, have a high unpredictability factor and these continue to emerge and spread across the globe, leading to global pandemics similar to the one affecting the population currently, the novel coronavirus. These diseases have a huge potential for damage and loss of life and are converting into epidemic proportions. Further, the absence of specific treatment options and frequent viral mutations have created panic among humankind. The globe is becoming increasingly interconnected, with globalisation a major trend in recent years, and this offers viruses further scope to affect global populations and evolve into life-threatening pandemics. Zoonotics are extremely dangerous as they cause high mortality and morbidity and also wreak havoc on public health systems, especially in developing and under-developed economies. Further, they also lead to significant economic losses in such countries. Loss of trade, tourism and consumer confidence are major aftereffects of global pandemics similar to COVID. In fact, reports peg the cost of 2003 SARS virus on the world economy at over 50 billion Us dollars.

Humanity has already been afflicted by dangerous pathogens and epidemics including plague, cholera, Middle East respiratory syndrome coronavirus, flu, and severe acute respiratory syndrome coronavirus or SARS-CoV. These diseases have originated due to increased contact with animals during breeding, hunting, and consumption. Considering the case of the coronavirus variants, these viruses belong to the Coronaviridae family and consist of four genera, namely alpha-, beta-, gamma-, and delta-coronaviruses. These viruses are enveloped, positive-sense, single-stranded, RNA viruses that cause infection in a wide range of animals and humans. Affected humans depict seasonal respiratory diseases, with alpha coronavirus genus HCoV-229E and HCoV-OC43 causing common colds and beta viruses such as HCoV-NL63 and HCoV-HKU1 causing more severe infections of the upper and lower respiratory tracts.

While studying the SARS-CoV Epidemic, it was found that this variant originated in China's Guangdong province in 2003, most likely through bats and palm civets. The 2002–2003 outbreak of SARS-CoV virus was reported in 29 countries belonging to North and South America, Europe and Asia and the case fatality rate stood at 9.7%. However, this virus depicted limited transmission rates and caused influenza-like syndromes with loose motions, fatigue and high fever. While patients depicted a number of symptoms, including pneumonia, the major cause of death was respiratory failure.

The MERS-CoV virus was reported ten years after the first case of the SARS-CoV. The new virus was discovered in Jeddah, Saudi Arabia and potential animal reservoirs included bats and dromedary camels. The disease spread to 27 countries and led to a total of at least 866 deaths, according to the World Health Organization. The variant led to symptoms such as mild to severe fulminant pulmonary disease, fever, chills, diarrhoea, headache, dry cough, arthralgia and myalgia, and was especially dangerous to people older than 65 years and people with comorbidities. Intermittent cases of the virus are still being reported and it is considered a threat to human health and potential. While vaccines are under development, clinical management of treatment includes supportive care for fever and pain, assistance to vital organ functions and treatment of secondary bacterial infections via antibiotics.

The latest variant from the Coronavirus family to affect humanity is the SARS-CoV-2 and infection from this virus has resulted in a globalpandemic. The infection originated in a cluster of patients in China's Wuhan region, in early December 2019 and the disease is now referred to as COVID-19. This infection is also, most likely, caused by bats but intermediary hosts are still being studied. While the infection is likely to be asymptomatic in almost 40% of the cases, the novel coronavirus causes symptoms ranging from mild fever, dry cough, shortness of breath, fatigue, nausea, diarrhoea, myalgia, weakness, etc. to pneumonia, acute liver injury, cardiac injury, kidney injury and neurologic illnesses. There is also a possibility of critically ill patients developing cytokine storms and macrophage activation syndrome.

The new coronavirus has wreaked havoc on the human health ecosystem by causing 14% to 19% of patients to be hospitalized, with 3% to 5% of patients requiring transfer to intensive care units following hypoxemic respiratory failures. Mortality of hospitalized patients is recorded at 15% to 20% and patients needing ICU intervention have depicted 40% fatality rates. Global mortality rates have been pegged between 0.25 and 3.0% according to Wilson N. et al., 2020, with higher rates seen in patients aged over 80 years. Children have depicted strong resistance to the infection with mild symptoms mostly limited to the upper respiratory tract.

According to the WHO dashboard on the COVID-19 pandemic, as of date, 20.4 crore confirmed cases have been reported across the globe, leading to a global death toll of 43.1 lakh deaths. Vaccination drives are underway, and the WHO reported that a total of 4.3 billion doses have been administered on a global scale. The Americas have the highest reported number of cases, followed by Europe, South-East Asia, Eastern Mediterranean, Africa and the Western Pacific region. The highest damage and loss of life has been reported in countries with developing economies and inadequate public health systems as well as regions with a large population aged 65 and above.

Chapter 2

COVID 19: Understanding Coronaviruses

Over the last one year, we have seen the global scientific and medical community come together and work tirelessly to envisage the right medical response to the ongoing COVID-19 pandemic. While we have met with some success, the larger question is, 'How do we nip such viruses in the bud?". The key lies in first understanding these unique animal viruses, studying their origins, and identifying key transmission routes.

2.1 What is a Coronavirus?

Coronaviruses are a family of viruses that cause diseases in mammals and birds. In humans, seven different types have been found, four of which are responsible for mild respiratory diseases. The common cold has originated from a mild version of a coronavirus. It was first discovered in 1965. The other three are known to cause more severe illnesses. SARS-CoV was responsible for SARS which affected China in 2002-2003 and spread to 28 countries and claimed 774 lives by 2003. MERS-CoV was responsible for MERS which broke out in Saudi Arabia in 2012. It was deadlier than SARS but less contagious – it killed 858 people. In 2019, SARS-Cov2 brought the COVID-19, which is considered more contagious than SARS, but has milder symptoms. However, since it is more widespread than any of the others, up to date the global death tally is over 4.3 million.

Exhibit 4: Corona viruses have been a part of human history

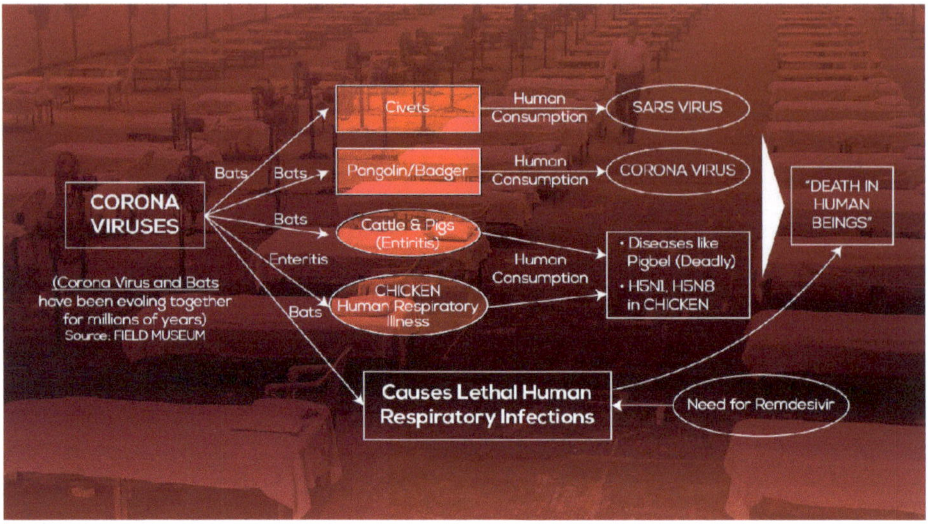

The coronaviruses are very small, about a tenth of a millimetre in size. They are spherical and coated with spikes of protein. In fact, they get their name 'corona' (Latin for crown) from the way they look and the crown like spikes around them. These spikes are what help the virus bind to healthy cells. Beneath these spikes is a membrane which can be disrupted by soap or alcohol, which is why washing your hands and using sanitizer are very effective in fighting the virus.

Inside the membrane is a genetic coding called RNA. RNA is very similar to DNA, but unlike DNA, RNA is single-stranded. They are constantly changing, which is responsible for the many variations of the virus. A viral test tells you if you have the virus in your system. The standard way to test whether you have the virus is by detecting if you have the nucleic acid by real-time reverse transcription polymerase chain reaction (rT-PCR).

Symptoms of COVID 19 include, but are not limited to, fever, dry cough, headache, fatigue, breathing difficulties, and loss of smell and taste. Symptoms vary depending on severity of the infection. The virus is strong in the sense that it has mutated several times, so symptoms vary depending from individual to severity of the case. Symptoms begin to appear 1 to 14 days after exposure. However, at least a third of the people do not develop noticeable symptoms. About 81% of cases are mild to moderate; 14% are severe (dyspnea, hypoxia) while 5% are critical (respiratory failure, shock, or multiorgan failure).

Mortality rates, even though fairly low (less than 1% for the age group under 65), are higher for older persons, ranging from 2.5% to 28% between the ages from 65 to 85. This is why the fight has been the strongest to protect the aged and highly at-risk population. People that have pre-existing conditions such as hypertension, diabetes, and cardiovascular diseases are more at risk from the coronavirus.

Like other pandemics, the COVID 19 pandemic came in waves as well. This happened mainly due to human behaviour. It also depends on the restrictions put forth by nations around the world and how diligent people were about following protocol of maintaining hygiene by washing their hands frequently, physical distancing and mask wearing. There is a clear correlation between areas where people were not following these practices and rising cases.

The 'first wave' brought about a soaring increase in infection which subsequently plateaued and started decreasing. Slowly, nations after educating their population about COVID and the protocol to follow, eased restrictions. Lockdowns opened up, communities opened up, restaurants, malls and bars restarted and people were understandably keen to get out. This is all the virus needed to breakout again.

For a few weeks, it wasn't noticeable. It took some time for people to start developing symptoms again and falling ill. Before long, cases were on the rise alarmingly again. The second wave came much deadlier and stronger than the first one. It was far more devastating than the first one. Looking back at previous pandemics, the second waves tend to be the worst.

Healthcare professionals are working tirelessly to find a cure to COVID 19, and vaccines have been produced worldwide and governments are working to get their population immunized at the earliest, but even today the primary way to keep safe is prevention. Management of the disease involves treating the symptoms, supportive care, and isolation for 14 days after the symptoms are first noticed.

2.2 How did it originate?

The virus is thought to originate from animals. The exact origination of patient zero is still unclear, however, there are several theories for the same and the investigation is ongoing. The consensus is that SARS-Cov2 originated sometime between October to November 2019. The first confirmed case was identified in the Wuhan province in China. However, we cannot be sure of the same. There are reports of it being circulated in Guangdong before Wuhan. One Italian study by the Italian National Cancer Institute claims it was found in Italy as of September 2019. The study found that there were 4 cases that tested positive for antibodies at the time.

The first announcement was made by Wuhan Municipal Health Commission on 31st December 2019, confirming 27 cases of an unknown pneumonia outbreak. This was alarming enough to start an investigation. A number of these people worked at a seafood market in Wuhan. At the time, human to human contact was not confirmed.

Experts believe that the virus had its origins in bats. That was the origin of MERS and SARS as well. It is theorised that the virus made the transmission to humans in one of China's wet markets which sold exotic wild animals such as cobras and wild boars. However, at the time of the outbreak, the wet markets were not selling bats. Therefore, the jump is thought to be made via a pangolin.

Exhibit 5: Bat viruses

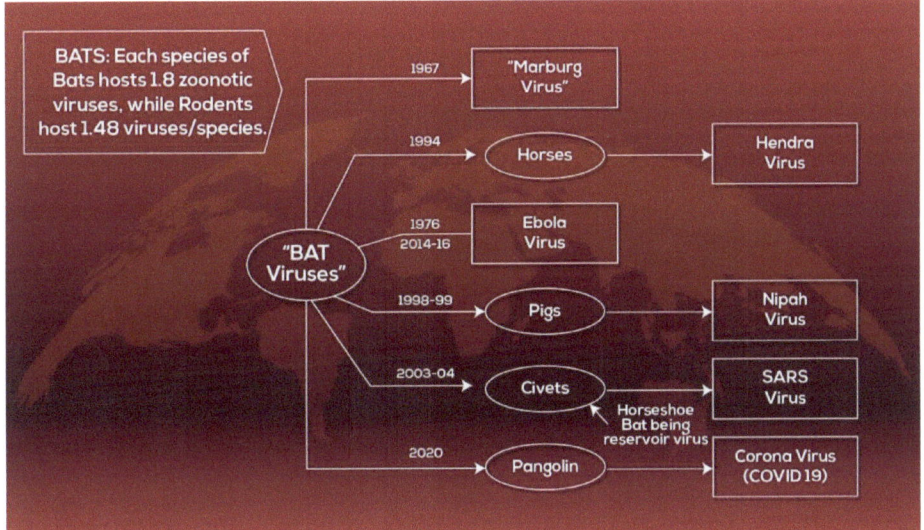

Human to human transmission was confirmed in January 2020 by the WHO due to the fact that people who had no direct contact with the animals, had started falling ill. By mid-January, the disease had already spread to nearby provinces in China. The official count of the infections at the time was 140 people, but now we know it was closer to 6000 people that had developed symptoms, and possibly many more infections. At this point, protective equipment was recommended for health professionals. On 30th January 2020, it was declared a Public Health Emergency. The spread factor was 100 to 200 at this point.

On February 21st 2020, Italy declared it's first case and within a month overtook China as the country with the most deaths due to COVID 19. Soon after, the United States overtook Italy and China with the highest number of confirmed cases. The virus was rapidly spreading across the world disrupting life as we know it. As of March 11th 2020, the WHO declared COVID 19 a global pandemic.

The national responses by countries across the world have been varied. Lockdowns were implemented by many countries restricting the movement and interactions of people. Governments were encouraging people to socially distance themselves. Terms like 'Stay at home' and 'Social distancing' became very common. The first lockdown was implemented in Wuhan in January 2020. Videos surfaced where Wuhan was a ghost-town and soon enough, the world followed suit.

Many countries have imposed travel bans, entry restrictions, quarantine facilities before travellers could enter the country, etc. The WHO has been the leading organisation taking charge of the world response. It has been heavily criticized in responding late to the coronavirus and it is believed that the WHO was caught between member nations and didn't perform as efficiently as it should have under the circumstances. An independent committee has been set up to examine the way that WHO responds to such public health emergencies.

As of August 2021, 205 million cases have been confirmed worldwide and the top 10 worst affected countries in order, are as follows: United States, India, Brazil, Russia, France, United Kingdom, Turkey, Argentina, Colombia, and Spain.

2.3 How is it Transmitted?

Human to human contact spreads in several ways. The most common way it can spread is if someone comes in contact with an infected person and liquid particles which are expended when a person speaks, coughs, sneezes, or breathes are exchanged.

It is now known that the virus spreads through close contact with an infected person. Close contact is defined as 1 meter or 3 feet. A person can get infected if the liquid particles come in contact with their eyes, nose, and mouth. The virus can also spread faster in poor ventilated environments, where the droplets tend to linger in the air for longer and could possibly transmit longer than 1 meter. People may also become infected by touching contaminated surfaces and then touching their eyes, nose or mouth.

Once infected, a person may start showing symptoms anytime between 1 to 14 days of incubation. However, the presence of symptoms does not have any bearing on how contagious the person is. All infected persons can spread the virus to other people, meaning that even if someone is asymptomatic, they could still spread the virus to people they come in contact with.

Data suggests that people seem to be the most infectious right from 2 days before they start developing symptoms. They stay contagious for a period of 14 days. Although, people with a more severe infection could remain infectious for a longer time.

Any event where people are closer to each other in proximity, there is a higher chance of the virus spreading and increases the chance of transmission. Large gatherings were the first to be banned by most nations, in the fear that they would turn into 'super spreader' events. Indoor locations with poor ventilation could be potential breeding grounds for transmission. There is also greater risk in activities where particles are expelled from the mouth, such as sports, heavy breathing, and singing.

Nations advised their citizens to avoid crowded places, maintain at least 1 meter distance from each other, keep their homes and spaces well ventilated, keep hands clean, sanitize or wash their hands for 30 seconds frequently, and wear a mask in public places. Big events with crowding were curtailed, weddings and funerals were allowed with a limited number of people; sporting events were held in isolation if not stopped completely; offices were closed down, 'work from home' was widely promoted especially for work that did not need physical presence. Digital connections soared and video meetings became a frequent occurrence. People were encouraged to stay at home if they felt even slightly unwell.

The protocol once you tested positive was to quarantine yourself at home and stay in a room away from your family. Quarantining oneself is the only way to contain it from spreading around you. If you come close to other people, mandatory 6 feet distancing and wearing a mask is strongly advised and enforced by law in a lot of countries. Governments built quarantine centres for people who did not have a place to quarantine. Since the start of the pandemic, medical facilities worldwide have been overwhelmed.

2.4 What makes it so Resilient?

The coronavirus is barely considered 'alive'. As soon as it enters a human system, it starts multiplying to create many more versions of itself. Before the person even has any symptoms, the virus has spread passing on to others. For now, we have no way to stop it.

It affects the nose, throat and can be more deadly when it affects the lungs. That's where the disease can kill. However, most of the time it stays in the upper respiratory tract, so that it can be coughed or transmitted to someone else easily. Since its symptoms are fairly mild, it passes on from person to person even before the host realises that he has it.

All viruses change with time and as they spread. Every time the COVID 19 virus inhabits a new host, it changes just a little bit. These changes are called mutations. A virus with multiple mutations is called a 'variant'. This is the main reason that COVID-19 has remained so resilient. There is no known singular treatment for COVID 19. We are still treating the symptoms more than the disease. Due to its several mutations, it is unpredictable and different individuals respond differently to it.

As the virus mutates, the symptoms change slightly. The virus mutates over borders, certain countries end up having a variant that is more deadly and some that is more contagious. So far, the variants of concern are: Alpha (originated in the United Kingdom), Beta (originated in South Africa), Gamma (originated in Japan/Brazil) and Delta (originated in India). Each variant spreads more rapidly than the last and could potentially be more severe.

Experts also claim that it will be nearly impossible to eradicate COVID 19. Vaccines will not be able to eliminate it. For eradication, infected persons will have to transmit it to less than one person on average. Early pandemic, one person was infecting at least 3, so we would have to immunize 60-70% of the population to achieve herd immunity. However, vaccines will not be able to stop transmission completely, they will just prevent symptoms. Thus, the virus will keep spreading. Although natural infection also provides immunity, it reduces risk of reinfection by

83% for a period of 5 months only. Therefore, reinfection after 5 months is likely, meaning that this virus is here to stay.

The next option is disease elimination, meaning that there would be zero new cases in an area for a sustained time period. Countries like New Zealand achieved this for a long-time using lockdown and border closure and diligent citizens doing their part. But keeping this up over the long run has proved to be impossible as people get more frustrated while cooped up indoors and with restrictions.

Immunization will be successful until a point. It will prevent severe cases, maybe even hospitalization and death but will not rule out infection entirely. Moreover, it will take a long time to immunize the whole world population. Not everyone feels as comfortable taking a relatively untested vaccine. (vaccines usually are tested over years to see their effectiveness and side effects). There are a growing number of people who don't want to take it despite the consequences for our population as a whole. Immunizing the world's population will also take time and be a large undertaking for all the nations.

Chapter 3

COVID 19: Why Can't I Eat Beef, Chicken or Pork, Please?

3.1 Eating Habits and Diseases

Most of us have been dependent on non veg diets for proteins. However, humans are not designed by nature to consume animals. The Covid 19 pandemic has been devastating. It has killed nearly 3 million people around the world and spread to over 220 countries. The virus has come from the human consumption of a bat infected mammal (Pangolin/Badger). Not from a laboratory in Wuhan! Dr. Embark's recent WHO trip confirms this. "Coronavirus likely came from a Mammal, not from a Laboratory" (Page, WSJ, Feb 9) helps validate the above. Dr. Rasmussen at Georgetown's piece in Nature Medicine corroborates this. We have to solve the "Correct Problem" first! Delve into the causes of SARS(2003), MERS (2012/13).

Exhibit 6: Eating habits and diseases

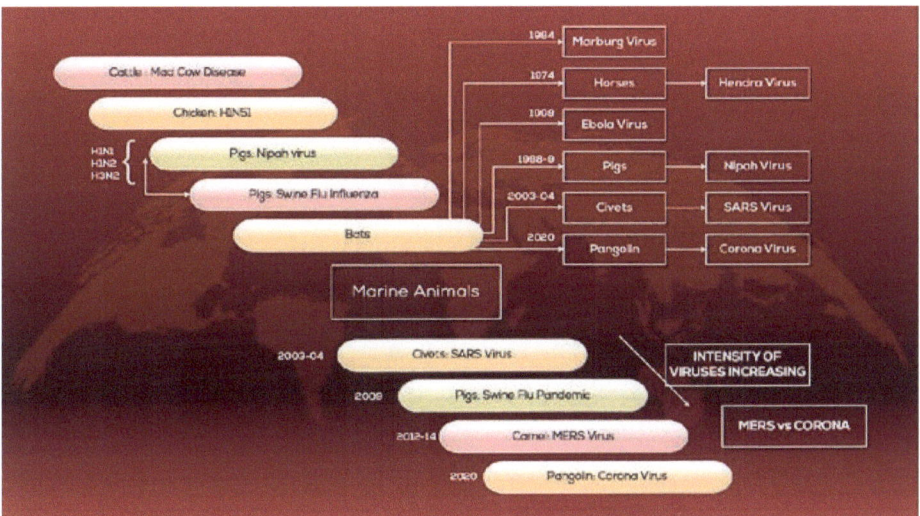

Animal viruses have been driven by human consumption of animals for the last 100 years. (Mad Cow Disease: Human consumption of Cattle) (H5N1: CHICKEN). (Avian Flu in China, 1959: Ducks) (Nipah Virus: Pigs) (Source: CDC) (SADS Disease: Pigs), (Swine Flu Pandemic,2009: Pigs) (Bats: Ebola Virus). As shown above, bats have been the intermediate host for both SARS and MERS.

Why can't we get rid of Bats? Bats are an integral part of the animal ecosystem; they pollinate over 500 plants and kill and eat toxic mosquitoes.

What we eat has always had a direct impact on both, our ability to stave off diseases and fight diseases. Food makes up the basic element of our nutrition and it is nutrition which ensures that the human body is capable of fighting off infections. It is very commonly said that a person is what he or she consumes and there is no doubt that a person's diet impacts their health, in positive and negative ways, depending on the constituent elements of the diet. Healthy eating habits can have a range of benefits for the human body, from the prevention of lifestyle diseases such as obesity and diabetes, to enhancing the psychological health of the body by improving mood and, in turn, the ability and desire to be active and physically fit.

A nutrient rich diet also supports the body by keeping the different parts fit and healthy. For instance, a calcium rich diet ensures that the person's bones remain strong and elastic. A diet rich in calcium and other minerals prevents osteoporosis while consuming unsaturated fats keeps the heart healthy and cardiovascular diseases at bay. Conversely, a high fat diet consisting of unhealthy fats can cause high blood pressure and a rise in cholesterol, posing threats to the heart. Consuming food items full of sugar, fat and calories can cause a number of diseases including strokes, heart attacks, type 2 diabetes, etc. Further, a heavy and unhealthy diet can also lead to tremendous weight gain and consequent burden on bones and joints, making the body weak and ungainly. With additional weight, internal organs are also forced to work harder, leading to untimely wear and tear and a number of health issues as time progresses.

A healthy diet also boosts immunity, helping individuals combat incoming diseases and also fight off infections. Consuming sufficient quantity of nutrients as part of a varied diet can help maintain the health and functioning of all human cells, including immune cells. Dietary patterns involving the consumption of probiotics, prebiotics and vitamins can ensure that the human body is primed to fight off microbial attacks and excess inflammation, making the immunity stronger and more robust even in the face of viral attacks. Each part of the body's immune cycle requires a number of micronutrients and therefore, consuming a well-rounded diet is necessary to maintain a healthy immune system. Nutrients such as vitamins C and D, iron, selenium, zinc, and protein have been identified as necessary elements for the growth and optimal function of immune cells.

3.2 Diseases Germinating from Food

Nowadays, it is becoming increasingly clear that certain diseases can actually germinate from the food we eat. It is a well-known fact that infectious organisms, including pathogenic protozoans, bacteria, and viruses have the ability to mutate and infect another host, despite being adapted to a particular animal host in the beginning of its lifecycle. While there are several instances of infectious agents in animal hosts altering themselves to infect human beings, such cases have not been seen in plant viruses. One of the most dangerous infectious agents at work against the human body is the ubiquitous virus and humankind has been in an age-old war with the agent.

As vehicles of gene transfer and promoters of host evolution, viruses have wreaked havoc on human bodies given their ability to learn from human immune systems. Several of the viruses which have recently attacked humankind, including SARS, MERS and SARS-CoV-2, belong to the RNA variant and these viruses possess extraordinary abilities to mutate, altering their genes and jumping the species barrier to widen their range of victims. With this innate capability to transform itself based on the host body, such viruses find it extremely easy to move from animals to human beings, and one of the major ways this happens is through ingestion. In fact, the eating habits of human beings have caused a number of preventable epidemics as well as an array of ailments in different parts of the body. In addition, environment sustainability is also enhanced by the consumption of plant-based food items.

Reports and experts hold that human beings consume more meat than is good for the human body and it is believed that a largely plant based diet would be much better for the overall human ecosystem. When talking about the 2002 SARS virus, most of the individuals who caught the diseases in the initial stages of the infection were known to have lived near live produce markets and quite a few of them were known food handlers with excessive exposure to animals. The SARS virus was finally traced to a palm civet, a raccoon dog, and a Chinese ferret-badger and, it was through these hosts that the virus infected the human beings working in the live animal markets in China's Shenzen municipality. In this instance, the SARS virus managed a jump from bats to the above-mentioned animals, and then moved on to human beings, leading to a major epidemic claiming several lives.

3.3 Coronaviruses Transferring to Different Animals

According to top virologists, Dr. Stanley Perlman and Anthony Fehr, "Coronaviruses: a review of their Replication and Pathogenesis" (National Library of Medicine)- Coronaviruses cause a variety of diseases in mammals and birds, ranging from Enteritis in cows and pigs, upper respiratory disease and kidney disease in chickens to potentially lethal human respiratory infections. These findings are from the top virologists in the world.

- Humans eating cattle, chickens, and pigs are causing these respiratory infections as the virus moves from animals to humans. Hence all the acute respiratory-related problems (similar to SARS). Hence the need for Oxygen. Hence the need for Remdesivir. If you do not eat these animals, you will not contract

these viruses. Regardless, we still continue to eat Beef, Chicken, and Pork.
- Coronavirus caused Enteritis in Pigs (Perlman, Fehr). It causes a life-threatening disease among people (particularly children) of the highlands of Papua New Guinea. This is caused by consumption of contaminated pig meat- caused by Clostridium Welchii Type C (an organism not usually present in the human intestine. Similar cases have been reported in Uganda and Thailand (Source: National Library of Medicine, PMID 575409).
- University of Chicago Booth/Columbia Study: 8% of US COVID cases from meatpacking plants, and contributing to nearly 5250 deaths by March 2020.
- Cohen in Science "Chinese pigs found to have human pandemic potential".

3.4 High Risk Food Groups

While the SARS virus jumped from animals to human beings in the live produce market, the consumption of infected animals also leads to people catching the disease and causing a pandemic as unprecedented as the current COVID outbreak. Considering the inherent risk in certain food groups, beef, chicken, and pork are known to be the most dangerous. Recent outbreaks of the COVID-19 infection at abattoirs and meat cutting plants in Germany have caused panic among individuals. Reports state that the virus affected employees at livestock facilities more than any other sector. While the lack of social distancing given the high capacity of such plants is one reason, there is also a strong possibility that the virus affected people because of their close contact with the high risk food groups such as beef, pork and chicken.

While it is stated that the virus cannot spread through meat that is well cooked on a high flame, there is a high likelihood of the virus spreading from a host animal to human beings through the consumption of raw or under-cooked meat. Since viruses require a host body to latch on to, it is important to complete a thorough cooking process, lasting at least 30 minutes, to kill the germs and viruses which may be present in the meat. Further, cross contamination is another possibility when it comes to the high risk food groups. This means that, in a kitchen, if a well-cooked dish is kept in contact with a raw or under-cooked one, there is a strong possibility of the cooked dish getting infected through the contact. Therefore, good hygiene is imperative when it comes to avoiding cross contamination and subsequent infection. Rigorous cleaning and consistent disinfection can help reduce the risk of contamination in raw food items.

What is the reason behind these food groups posing such high risk? Not only are these food groups adept vectors for viral infections, they also carry a number of other disease-causing germs within themselves. In fact, many of the diseases affecting human beings are directly linked to domestic meat species of beef, pork, lamb, and poultry. Such diseases include everything from E. coli to salmonella. Category wise, ground beef is a known source of E. coli while beef cattle cause bovine spongiform encephalitis or BSE. Pork is known to cause trichinosis and poultry causes salmonella. Additionally, the meat and poultry industry is vulnerable to a number of infectious diseases that may erupt in food processing areas, as seen at the abattoirs in Germany. Such situations become the breeding grounds for foodborne infections like salmonella and trichinosis, caused by consuming food that is contaminated with bacteria, parasites, and viruses. Two of the particularly dangerous foodborne bacteria are clostridium botulinum, which is known to develop in vacuum-packaged and canned foods, and listeria monocytogenes, which is seen in spaces with poor cleaning of machines, unclean floors and dirty drains.

Considering the risk factor inherent in beef, the food group can cause BSE, or mad cow disease, which is a deadly brain-degenerative illness in cattle. The disease causes a spongy deterioration of the brain and the spinal cord and has a long incubation period of up to eight years, making it difficult to detect it in cattle. It affects all species and is known to jump from cattle to humans who consume food contaminated by the brain, spine or digestive system of the infected animal. In recent times, severe outbreaks of BSE have crippled the Canadian beef export industry. The disease, which manifests as the Creutzfeldt-Jakob disease in human beings, has also affected people in the United Kingdom and other meat-eating countries.

The common infection agent E. coli is another bacterium found in the intestines of human beings and animals. While the bacterium is not considered parasitic within the food tract, if it gains access to organs such as the kidneys, bladder or other internal organs, it is known to turn parasitic and cause fatal infections. E. coli outbreaks are also mostly associated with beef, especially ground meat supplies. Salmonella, the infectious agent present in poultry, causes typhoid fever in human beings. Raw or undercooked pork can lead to the possibility of catching trichinosis, a foodborne infection causing nausea, diarrhoea, vomiting, fatigue, fever, and abdominal discomfort.

3.5 Increased Vulnerability to Viruses

Viruses are, undoubtedly, a major threat to the human population, and high risk food groups such as beef, pork and chicken contribute to the spread of such dangerous viruses. Viruses present in food, which cause foodborne diseases such as the ones described above, are a cause of concern for public health and well-being and require special attention as they are significantly different from bacteria which can be easily treated through the prescription of antibiotics. Further, there is a lack of effective virus contamination measures, leading to an amplification of symptoms and infection each time a new virus or variant presents itself.

Recent studies and surveys have indicated that foodborne viral infections are extremely common in various parts of the globe and the situation is further worsened because of under-reporting, lack of surveillance systems and the inability of existing systems to determine the number and proportion of illnesses being transmitted by foodborne channels in comparison with other common routes. This makes it tough to estimate the proportion of viral diseases which are foodborne. Considering the clear dissimilarities in the morphology, infectivity, persistence and epidemiology between viruses and the common foodborne bacteria, it becomes more difficult for risk managers to assess the risk factor inherent within high risk food groups such as beef, pork and poultry.

Another factor to consider is the aspect that regular consumption of such high risk food items could also weaken the human body and immune system internally. For instance, high consumption of red meat and fatty pork can cause obesity in human being and this makes the human body more susceptible to viral attacks. Additionally, obesity could also cause co-morbidities such as high blood pressure and high cholesterol, which makes the human body more vulnerable in pandemic situations. Consumption of meat produce also puts more strain on the digestive system and internal organs which need to work harder to process the food when compared to a light plant-based diet.

Plant-based diets have also been known to lower risks of strokes and keep the brain healthy, in addition to helping maintain good levels of cholesterol. Risk of type 2 diabetes is also lowered by the consumption of a plant-based diet. Therefore, a plant-based diet is a better option to keep the human body healthier, indicating that a meat-based diet, which is heavily dependent on the consumption of high-risk food groups such as beef, pork, and chicken, could lead to increased vulnerabilities in the human body. These vulnerabilities are not limited to just lifestyle diseases but also to the outbreak of pandemics and infectious foodborne diseases which cause loss of health as well as untimely and unwarranted deaths.

COVID 19: Why Can't I Eat Beef, Chicken or Pork, Please? | 47

Exhibit 7: Human consumption of animals is devastating the ecosystem

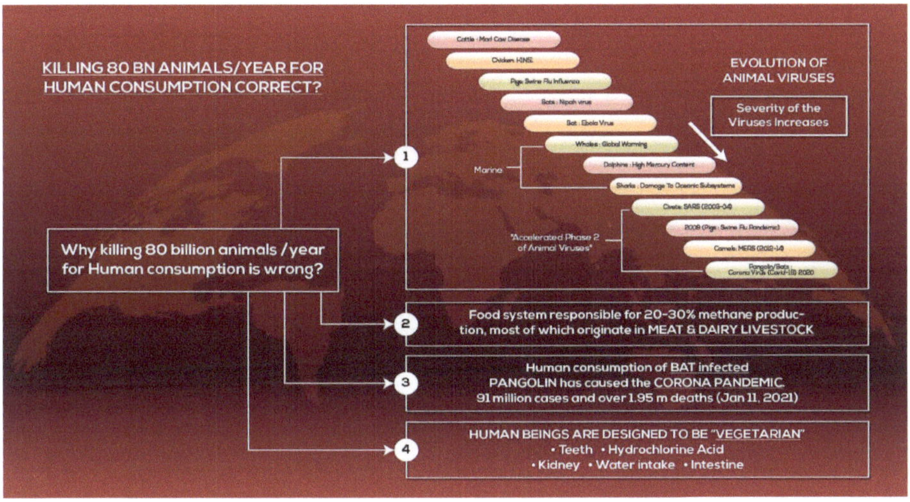

KILLING 80 BN ANIMALS/YEAR FOR HUMAN CONSUMPTION CORRECT?		EVOLUTION OF ANIMAL VIRUSES
	Cattle : Mad Cow Disease	
	Chicken : H1N1	
	Pigs : Swine Flu Influenza	Severity of the Viruses Increases
	Bats : Nipah virus	
	Bat : Ebola Virus	
	Marine — Whales : Global Warming	
	Dolphins : High Mercury Content	
	Sharks : Damage To Oceanic Subsystems	
	Civets: SARS (2003-04)	
	2009 (Pigs : Swine Flu Pandemic)	
	"Accelerated Phase 2 of Animal Viruses" — Camels: MERS (2012-14)	
	Pangolins/Bats, Corona Virus (Covid-19) 2020	

① Why killing 80 billion animals /year for Human consumption is wrong?

② Food system responsible for 20-30% methane production, most of which originate in MEAT & DAIRY LIVESTOCK

③ Human consumption of BAT infected PANGOLIN has caused the CORONA PANDEMIC. 91 million cases and over 1.95 m deaths (Jan 11, 2021)

④ HUMAN BEINGS ARE DESIGNED TO BE "VEGETARIAN"
• Teeth • Hydrochlorine Acid
• Kidney • Water intake • Intestine

Human beings and animals are different ecosystems. Human beings cannot encroach on the animal ecosystem. Period. Obey the "Design of Life".

Chapter 4

Wuhan & Why We Didn't Learn from SARS?

4.1 What happened in Wuhan?

The ongoing COVID pandemic broke out in late 2019 in Wuhan province of China and is now a global contagion endangering uncountable lives and businesses. Several studies have been made into the happenings in Wuhan which led to a pandemic of this unprecedented scale. There have been various questions around the occurrence. How did the virus spill over from bats to humans? Where did it originate? Is there any truth behind the conspiracy theories doing the rounds? There are many who believe that the virus leaked out of a Wuhan laboratory which was conducting active research on SARS strains of viruses. And then, there are worrisome theories about how the virus was genetically modified in the lab and then let out into the world. There have been countless debates and attempts at answering this all pervasive question. Where did the virus, which claimed the lives of scores of people across the globe, and pushed several people into abject poverty, originate and how did it make its way across the globe at such a frightening pace?

There have been multiple studies into the matter but, nobody can state for sure how the pandemic originated or where it came from. Everyone knows the first outbreak occurred in Wuhan but, how did the novel coronavirus reach Wuhan? And what are the events which led to the deadly outbreak? There are two distinct schools of thought governing the tragedy. The first believes that this is a natural zoonotic event which went on to gain in scale because of limited travel restrictions in the early days of the outbreak. There are a number of possibilities that support this theory – most realistically, the zoonotic jump could have occurred from bats to humans or it could have been facilitated by an intermediary host. This is exactly what happened during the previous SARS and MERS outbreaks. However, the concern lies in the fact that, despite the time that has passed, scientists have been unable to track the intermediary host which carried the ongoing coronavirus to the humans. In previous SARS outbreaks, the intermediary host was traced much sooner.

The second probable school of thought states that the virus escaped from the research laboratory in Wuhan which is known for studying and working with exactly this specimen of SARS. Later on in this book we delve further into why this theory is completely unsubstantiated and defies logic.

Keeping the theories aside, it was on December 31, 2019 that Wuhan Municipal Health Commission reported a cluster of pneumonia cases, leading to the eventual identification of the novel coronavirus. Even as the World Health Organization took efforts to contain the incident through management support teams and issued a comprehensive package of technical guidelines to advice countries on how to detect, test and manage potential cases, the first recorded case of COVID, outside China, was reported in Thailand on January 13, 2020. From there on, the virus metastasized into a global contagion affecting almost all countries and claiming lives and livelihoods across geographies.

Exhibit 8: Collective amnesia

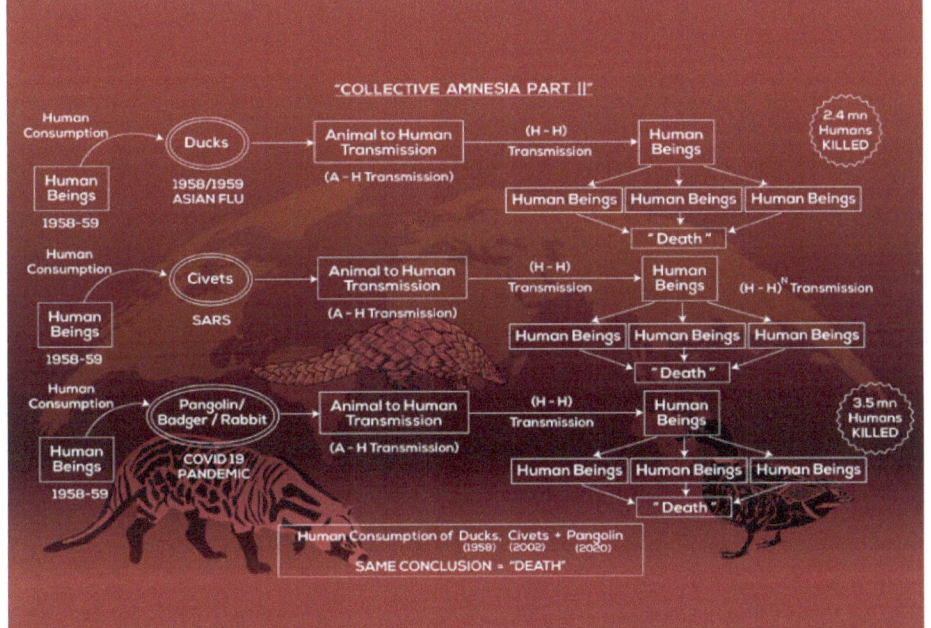

4.2 The Domino Effect!

While the pandemic began spreading its grasp across countries, economies began to go into lockdown to counter the outbreak. Death toll was rising, especially in the older population and individuals with co-morbidities and, with no sign of a vaccine on the horizon, people were scared to step out of their homes. Masks became ubiquitous and social gatherings grinded to a halt. Industries shut shops and companies which could function online moved their work to the digital platform. Work from home became a reality and only essential service providers were allowed to commute freely. Even within countries, regional boundaries were enforced and travel was discontinued except for the most emergent reasons.

The virus not only affected global health systems but global economies as a whole – supply chains shut down, leading to a pile up of demand and lack of supply. People lost jobs and their livelihoods. Spending dropped to dismal lows, pushing economic growth into unprecedented downturns even as inflation rose in essential items. People were affected mentally, physically and psychologically by the pandemic and cities saw mass exodus of residents who tried to return to the relative safety of their hometowns. Amidst all this, the virus spread like a wildfire, affecting families left, right and centre.

Technology providers had a field day with everyone from corporate employees to students reaching out for internet and connecting gadgets. Everything from work to school to family gatherings went online, putting tremendous pressure on the infrastructure in developing and underdeveloped countries. Healthcare systems struggled to cope with the onslaught of incoming cases and frontline workers were exhausted and burnt out. Several doctors and nurses lost their lives in the fight against the pandemic. Studies believe that this damaging domino effect could have been reduced significantly if only the response to the first outbreak had been more stringent. Countries kept their borders open and allowed travel and tourism in the early days of the virus, showing concern only when cases began to rise. With the virus once within geographical borders, it was difficult to contain it despite nationwide lockdowns, quarantines, and constraints on travel.

4.3 History Repeats Itself - SARS

China was the epicentre of another major epidemic, the SARS infection of 2002. A form of atypical pneumonia, SARS began spreading around the world in November 2002, pushing the WHO to name it a worldwide health threat. In China, the epidemic infected over 5,300 people and killed 349. The epidemic created China's greatest socio-political crisis since the 1989 Tiananmen Square massacre and economists believed that the Chinese economy would go into a severe downturn. Everything from the health and security of the Chinese people as well as the entire state of reform, development, and stability were put at risk, along with China's national interest and international image. Following months of stringent action, the Chinese government managed to control the infection, eliminating all known virus incidents by the middle of August 2003.

While the government failed to prevent the outbreak early on, subsequent mass mobilization ensured that the infection was successfully controlled. However, despite the 2002 outbreak, and advancements in the field, China was unable to prevent the outbreak of the ongoing pandemic. Studies suggest that, despite the strong action against SARS in 2002, China's ability to effectively prevent and contain future viruses was uncertain and the blame for this is placed on the fact that prevention and control programmes in the country with the world's largest population are still affected by problems in agenda-setting, policy making, and implementation. Governmental policies and a lack of transparency are considered to be the reasons for this dilemma.

4.4 What Happened at the Time of SARS?

Research and analysis suggests that China's health system responded relatively well to the initial outbreak of the SARS epidemic. The strange disease, discovered first in Foshan and then in Heyuan and Zhongshan in Guangdong, alerted Chinese health personnel to the incoming threat in mid-December 2002 and the new provincial government ordered an investigation around January 20, 2003 following various other steps taken by provincial and state authorities in the meantime. While a confidential report was dispatched to the authorities by January 27, 2003 further response was delayed by a lack of information flow and transparency within the Chinese hierarchy. The public and most health workers were uninformed about the disease since the report was largely kept under wraps and only released as a bulletin to the frontline workers, most of whom were on vacation owing to the Chinese New Year celebrations taking place across the country.

Further, the report was classified as a state secret, preventing caregivers from sharing details with the public. The information blackout continued till February. The silence was finally broken by Guangdong health officials who held press conferences on February 11, admitting there were no effective drugs to treat the disease and stating that the outbreak was only tentatively contained. With the restrictions on information and awareness campaigns, the Chinese population was unable to protect itself from the outbreak, leading to mass chaos and dissatisfaction with the government. The governmental inaction, combined with the absence of an effective response to the initial outbreak resulted in a crisis.

The mistakes we made

COVID reached India on January 27, 2020, when a woman was admitted to a Kerala hospital complaining of dry cough and sore throat. While residents were advised to wear masks and practice social distancing, a nationwide lockdown was only mandated on March 24, allowing the virus time to spread across state borders. Even as the state and central governments took steps to mitigate the fallout from the pandemic, the first and second waves of COVID have wreaked havoc across India's socio-economic milieu. Several mistakes have been made, with the government under blame for inadequate action and delayed responses. Reports state that the government's COVID-19 taskforce had not met in months prior to the second wave in April 2021.

The Indian government claimed, in 2020, to have beaten the virus with a relatively low mortality rate, despite multiple warnings regarding the potential dangers of a second wave and the emergence of a new variant. Super-spreader events were allowed and the authorities maintained that the country was safe. The vaccination policy was also understaffed and unprepared to cater to the over billion-strong population in the country, creating further distress among the affected masses. The central government was blamed for not conducting adequate discussions with the state governments and for the severe outbreak in the second wave, which resulted in several unwarranted deaths. Termed a self-inflicted catastrophe, India's response to the second wave was disparaged across the globe.

What we Should Have Learnt?

The global pandemic has put forth several lessons that countries should have learnt and assimilated from previous such events. The importance of steps including the early detection of outbreaks, transparent and effective communication in the event of an outbreak, the promotion of research and development, strategies for containment, and multinational collaboration in implementing such strategies have been discussed time and again. Surveillance and containment are the first steps in response to any viral crisis, and countries must strengthen national capacities for surveillance, response, and control of future communicable diseases. While laboratories must be established to study and counter potential threats, it is also essential to maintain absolute safety in such spaces to avoid possible leaks in the future. Further, surveillance must be followed by action and reinforced with adequate laboratory capacity, skilled and well-trained professionals, as well as a legal structure focused on transparency, global cooperation, and public protection.

Studies state that about 75% of emerging human pathogens and 61% of all human pathogens are zoonotic and it is imperative that governments across the globe collaborate to create a war-chest against future infections of this scale. With animal markets creating a fertile breeding ground for future viruses, it is also essential to ensure utmost cleanliness in such dangerous zones. Work on vaccines and anti-viral therapies should be expanded to counter threats arising in the future. Countries should stockpile broad-spectrum antiviral drugs, establish surge capacity for rapid vaccine production, and develop models to define the most effective channel of delivering medical care in the event of viral outbreaks. Quarantine centres and home quarantine capabilities should be developed, in tandem with educating the public and building trust in health authorities, compensating quarantined workers and offering incentives to health care and frontline workers.

The media and expert professionals should be included in counter measures. They should be channelized to inform the public at the outset of a pandemic and a structure should be created to empower people and help them manage panic and anxiety in the face of an unprecedented crisis.

Chapter 5

Understanding [(A-H) + (H-H) Raise to N] Transmission

5.1 Dynamics of COVID-19 = Same as the Asian Flu Pandemic (1959) & SARS

ANIMAL VIRUSES have been driven by the human consumption of animals for the last 80-100 years. The last century is peppered with several instances of transmission of animal viruses from animals to humans simply through the consumption of animals. Take for example, the Mad Cow Disease which was caused due to the human consumption of cattle or the H5N1 virus which stemmed from the human consumption of chicken. This mechanism of (Animal-Human) and (Human-Human Transmission) raise to N has been seen in the Asian Flu Pandemic of 1958/59 (human consumption of Ducks, see chart below), the SARS virus (human consumption of civets) as well as in the current pandemic which stemmed from the human consumption of pangolins, badgers, and rabbits. Please see the illustrative chart below.

The Killer Bat

Exhibit 9: Collective Amnesia Part 2

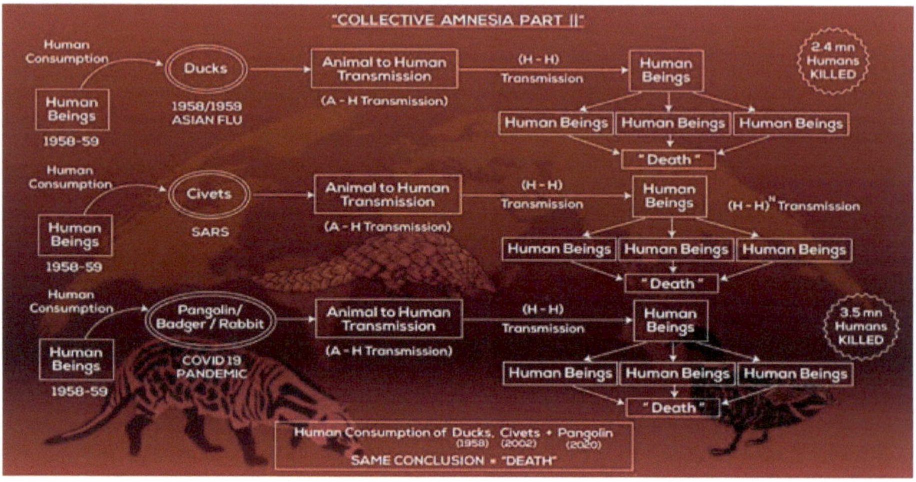

"COLLECTIVE AMNESIA PART II"

[Diagram showing three parallel flows:

Row 1: Human Consumption → Ducks (1958/1959 ASIAN FLU) → Animal to Human Transmission (A - H Transmission) → (H - H) Transmission → Human Beings → Human Beings | Human Beings | Human Beings → "Death" — 2.4 mn Humans KILLED. Human Beings 1958-59.

Row 2: Human Consumption → Civets (SARS) → Animal to Human Transmission (A - H Transmission) → (H - H) Transmission → Human Beings → (H - H)^N Transmission → Human Beings | Human Beings | Human Beings → "Death". Human Beings 1958-59.

Row 3: Human Consumption → Pangolin/Badger/Rabbit (COVID 19 PANDEMIC) → Animal to Human Transmission (A - H Transmission) → (H - H) Transmission → Human Beings → Human Beings | Human Beings | Human Beings → "Death" — 3.5 mn Humans KILLED. Human Beings 1958-59.

Human Consumption of Ducks, Civets + Pangolin (1958) (2002) (2020)
SAME CONCLUSION = "DEATH"]

Unfortunately, instances of such viruses are increasing both in numbers as well as intensity. For example, the deadly Avian Flu in 1959 in China (H2N2) virus was caused due to the human consumption of ducks. By the time the second wave had ended, the virus had infected between 250 million to a billion people and killed between 1-4 million people. While the name of the virus and the animal changes, the story remains the same. Same thing with SARS. Different Animal = Civets in SARS (2002/2003).

According to top virologists, Dr. Stanley Perlman and Anthony Fehr, "Coronaviruses: a review of their Replication and Pathogenesis" (National Library of Medicine)- Coronaviruses cause a variety of diseases in mammals and birds, ranging from Enteritis in cows and pigs to upper respiratory disease in chickens. These findings are from the top virologists in the world. The key variants are caused by the mega-multiplier effects of human consumption of these animals. Not from thin air. The schematic shown below explains the (H-H Transmission); (H-H Transmission) raise to N.

My hypothesis is that the Variant B1617 (India variant) is caused due to the human consumption of Chicken (please see the illustration shown below). There is Animal-Human Transmission (A-H) and then Human to Human (H-H Transmission) and then (Human-Human Transmission) raise to N. In that sense, such viruses ultimately have a domino effect on the population. This has happened with several animal viruses with (Human to Human Transmission) raise to N- Nipah (1997) Ebola

Understanding [(A-H) + (H-H) Raise to N] Transmission | 59

(Bats,1997 and 2013), Swine Flu Pandemic (2009) SARS (Civets, 2003), MERS (Camels, 2004) and now COVID 19.

Exhibit 10: Transmission from Animals to Humans

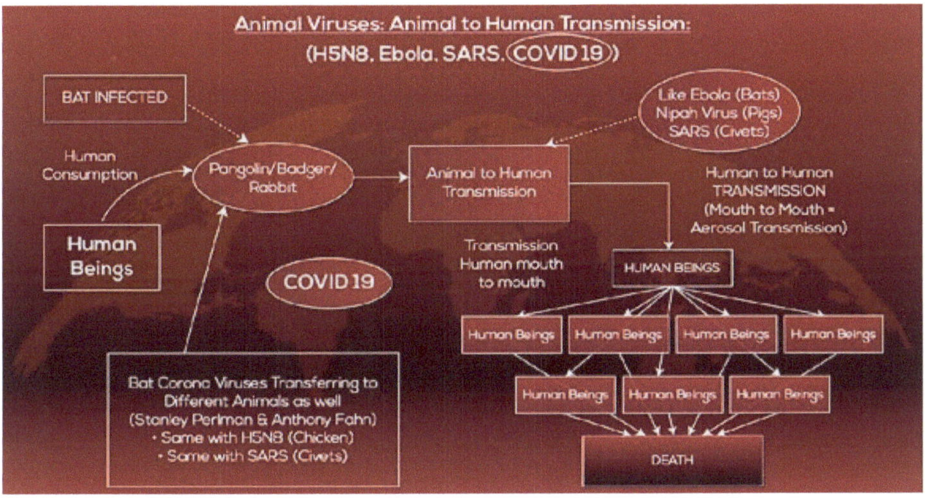

5.2 Network Effects of the Covid 19 Virus

The virus spreads from human mouth to mouth over very short distances (aerosol transmission). Not airborne over very short distances. This helps the virus spread faster.

Let's imagine a 'not so hypothetical' scenario.

A passenger who has consumed pangolin/badger in garlic sauce carries the virus. He then spreads it by sneezing or by aerosol transmission to 30 other passengers on the plane to New York or Iran or the United Kingdom (each), and then spreads it to another 40 people at the airport; each of the 70 people pass it on to 50 people each (being at a close distance), so 3500 people, each passes it on to 100 people each by being close to another human being through aerosol transmission.

So, now, 350,000 people have got the virus. As you can see, the virus does not spread in a linear fashion. Instead, it spreads exponentially. This is similar to "Network Effect" in Information Theory. The "scalability" of the virus is far greater than what we saw in the case of the SARS Virus. Much greater than SARS. By Design.

Exhibit 11: Devastating impact on Human Civilization

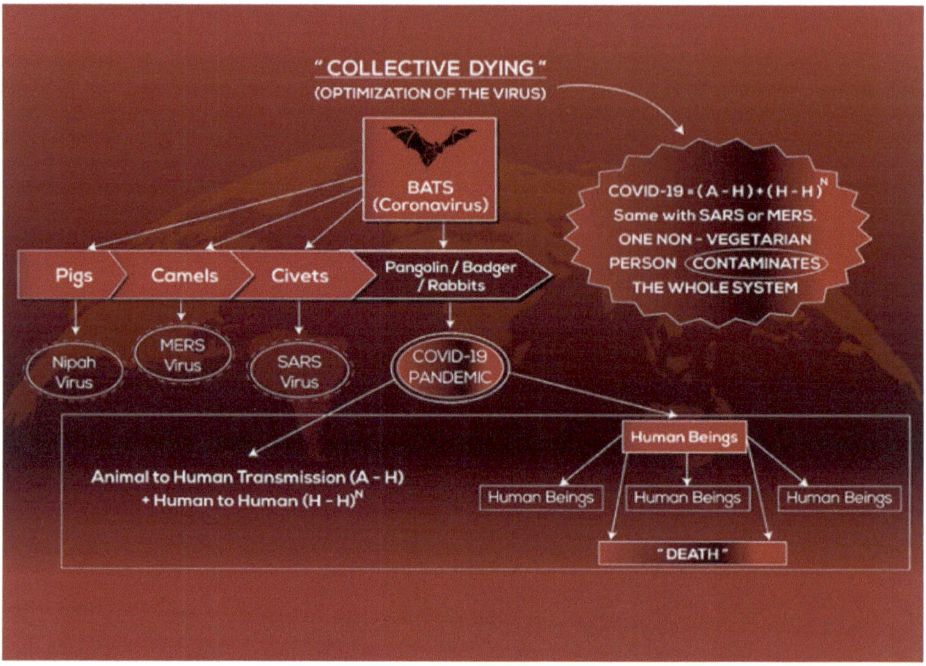

[Figure: Flow diagram titled "COLLECTIVE DYING" (OPTIMIZATION OF THE VIRUS), showing BATS (Coronavirus) transmitting to Pigs (Nipah Virus), Camels (MERS Virus), Civets (SARS Virus), and Pangolin/Badger/Rabbits (COVID-19 Pandemic), leading to Animal to Human Transmission (A–H) + Human to Human (H–H)^N, resulting in Human Beings "DEATH". Side note: COVID-19 = (A–H) + (H–H)^N. Same with SARS or MERS. ONE NON-VEGETARIAN PERSON CONTAMINATES THE WHOLE SYSTEM.]

5.3 "Optimization" of the Covid Virus

When getting a Masters in Operations Research at the world's No. 1 Operational Research and Industrial Engineering Program at Cornell University, I learned valuable lessons on linear programming, semidefinite programming, and combinatorial optimization to better understand the necessary rules governing "Optimization." One is always finding Minima and Maxima of functions, subject to so-called "constraints." When one thinks of the "Optimization of the Coronavirus,"= Aerosol transmission via human mouth to mouth transmission leading to a "Massive Multiplier" effect of the virus is close to optimal. This will inflict the "maximum" amount of damage to human beings. Basically, like SARS and MERS, it causes respiratory symptoms. Over 3 million human lives have been lost so far.

Bats have been the intermediate host for several viruses that the Hendra virus (Horses), Nipah virus (Pigs), MERS virus (Camels), SARS v(Civets), and now the COVID 19 virus (Pangolin/Badgers).

Human consumption of these animals, in turn, led to (Animal-Human) Transmission, and in many cases like in the Asian Flu, SARS and MERS led to (Human-Human) raise to N transmission. The schematic of Bats being the host of various viruses is illustrated in the chart shown below. Also, the human consumption of Bats in West Africa led to the deadly Ebola virus (Direct).

Chapter 6

COVID 19: Why the Lab Theory is Bogus!

The debate between whether the novel coronavirus was developed in a lab or was the outcome of natural selection has been raging since the first case was identified in late 2019 in Wuhan province of China. Take into account the fact that Wuhan is the site of major laboratories researching viruses belonging to the SARS family and conspiracy theories abound. Following considerable discussion and in-depth study into the matter, there are some aspects which have helped confirm the fact that the virus did not, conclusively, originate in a laboratory.

6.1 Natural Selection vs. Manipulation Theory

The novel coronavirus, also termed as the SARS-CoV-2, is the seventh coronavirus which has been identified as infectious agents affecting human beings. Of these seven variants, severe illnesses are caused by SARS-CoV, MERS-CoV and SARS-CoV-2 while the variants HKU1, NL63, OC43 and 229E cause only mild symptoms. A number of studies, across the virus spectrum, has indicated that the ongoing pandemic has not been manipulated or created in a laboratory but is, rather, a product of natural selection.

The new virus is highly contagious, which has prompted governments across the world to mandate lockdowns and enforce social distancing with the hope of limiting the spread. Affecting the human respiratory system and causing illnesses related to the Acute Respiratory Distress Syndrome, the new variant has greatly impacted human health and well-being on an unprecedented and global scale. Studies from the onset suggested that this virus would create a much larger impact on global health infrastructure and economy, when compared with other virus outbreaks of the same family. The higher infectiousness and rapid spread of the virus forced people to question the origin of the virus and wonder whether it was genetically manipulated to create extreme damage. Further, the fact that existing vaccines were not effective against the virus also caused people to believe that the virus was manipulated in a lab and then leaked into the unsuspecting populace.

Conspiracy theories also emerged from the fact that economic and trade related tensions were already brewing between America and China, the world's two most prosperous economies. People whispered that the virus was a way of making America weak and building upon China's stronghold over the global ecosystem. Separately, given that China was first affected by the pandemic, people also considered the possibility of America having created the virus and causing the leak to damage China's prosperity and global standing. The virus came to be considered as a potential weapon of biological warfare and spread fear in the minds of lay people who were already panicking given the rapid spread and lack of healthcare facilities or treatment options. What worsened the situation was the fact that news and social media platforms also amplified the message, making people believe in its veracity. Conspiracy theories always gain more supporters than scientifically proven facts and this adage was brought to fore with the fake news revolving around the virus.

6.2 Argument for Natural Selection

Multiple research studies suggest that there is no factual evidence in support of the laboratory manipulation theory. Genetic analyses of the novel coronavirus as well as related viruses do not indicate any possibility of genetic manipulation or bioengineering. In fact, the studies are stated to conclusively prove that the virus could not have originated in a lab, it could only be a product of natural selection. The study of the virus began shortly after the epidemic began, with Chinese scientists sequencing the genome of the virus and making the information available to worldwide scientists for further study and analysis. The study denoted that Chinese authorities had, in fact, ensured rapid detection of the virus and took preventive action but the virus kept transmitting through frequent human-to-human transmission following a single introduction into the human population.

The research shared by the Chinese scientists has been used by subsequent researchers to prove that the virus is, indeed, designed by natural selection and the tell-tale features of the virus have helped prove this fact. Studies have focused on the genetic template for the viral spike proteins on the outside of the virus, which are used to bind to cell surface receptors and facilitate entry into human host cells. Two important features of the spike protein – the receptor-binding domain and the spike's polybasic furin cleavage site – prove that the virus is a by-product of natural selection. The polybasic furin cleavage site is involved in the virus entering into the host cell's outer membrane, thus playing the role of a molecular can opener. Studies have pointed out that the receptor-binding domain of the new coronavirus is optimized for binding to human angiotensin-converting enzyme 2, leading to the infection, and such a feature is most likely the outcome of natural selection on a human or human-like ACE2 which allows the scenario to develop adequately and lead to major infections. This has been considered as verifiable proof of the virus' evolution through natural selection.

Further evidence for natural selection arises from a study of the virus' backbone or overall molecular structure. The evidence states that, if the virus was a product of bioengineering or genetic manipulation, the virus would have been created from the backbone of a strain known to cause illness. However, the backbone of the novel coronavirus differed significantly from the molecular structures of known viruses, greatly resembling similar viruses found in the bodies of bats and pangolins. This indicates that the new coronavirus is not a derivation from the backbone of any of the previously existing SARS virus strains. Therefore, these two distinct features, the mutations in the receptor-binding domain, and the distinctive backbone exhibited by the virus, helped scientists verify that the novel coronavirus, which has caused an unprecedented global pandemic, is not the result of a lab manipulation but rather the by-product of consistent natural selection.

6.3 Why is Manipulation not a Robust Theory?

Research and advanced studies state that the probability of the novel coronavirus arising from laboratory manipulation is extremely minute. While the afore-mentioned two reasons indicate natural selection, there is another loophole in the manipulation theory. Scientists state that, if manipulation was the factor, then one of the multiple reverse-genetic systems available for betacoronavirus would have been utilised to create the new variant. However, as we saw above, genetic data unequivocally states that the SARS-CoV-2 under study is not derived from any of the previously present virus backbones. There are two scenarios then, which can be the basis for the natural selection and evolution of the novel coronavirus.

Natural selection in an animal host prior to zoonotic transfer

Under this school of thought, there is a possibility that an animal source was present at the location of infection. This is largely probable when considering the Huanan market in Wuhan, which is known as a live produce centre trading in all varieties of animals. Considering the similar features of SARS-CoV-2 and the bat virus akin to SARS-CoV, there is a strong probability that bats in the live produce market acted as the reservoir hosts for the virus. Further, Malayan pangolins, which were illegally imported into the Guangdong province in China, also contain coronaviruses which are extremely similar to the novel virus which affected humankind. While the bat virus, scientifically termed RaTG13, is the closest in structure to the COVID virus, pangolin viruses have also exhibited strong similarity to the novel coronavirus, especially when considering the receptor-binding domain. This indicates that the SARS-CoV-2 spike protein was, indeed, optimized through hosts, for binding to human-like ACE2, verifying the likelihood of the virus having originated through natural selection. While no animal virus has yet been identified as the direct progenitor of the coronavirus under question, studies maintain that the diversity of coronavirus existing in bats and other animal species is yet highly under-analysed.

Natural selection in humans in the aftermath of zoonotic transfer

This theory holds that there is a possibility that a progenitor of the novel coronavirus jumped into humans from animal hosts and acquired genomic features through consecutive adaptations during unhindered and undetected human-to-human transmissions. Once the virus made its way into the human body, the subsequent adaptations enabled the pandemic to spread and create a significantly large cluster of cases, effectively triggering an outbreak which then metamorphosed into a global contagion. Studies into the timing of the most recent ancestor of the virus responsible for the ongoing pandemic indicate that the virus most probably emerged between late November 2019 and early December of the same year, which is also in line with the earliest retrospectively confirmed occurrences of the infection. This indicates a period of unidentified transmission among humans, the time period between zoonotic transmission and the development of the infection-causing polybasic cleavage sites. Similar was the case of the Middle Eastern Respiratory Syndrome Covid virus during which all human cases originated from zoonotic jumps via dromedary camels.

While the continued research on SARS virus in laboratories did prompt people to consider the possibility of a lab leak and genetic manipulation to create a bioweapon, the finding of similar viruses in bats and pangolins has created multiple loopholes in the conspiracy theory. In the same scenario, there is undeniable proof supporting the natural selection and evolution of the virus which has threatened the economic and physical well-being of a number of countries across the globe.

6.4 Lab Theory a Bogus Perception

The novel coronavirus has disrupted everything from human health to economic and social wellbeing, pushing people to consider all sorts of theories to understand the unprecedented and cataclysmic event. In the aftermath of the black swan event, it is natural that people would consider all sorts of possibilities regarding the evolution of the virus which has claimed many lives and destroyed the livelihoods of countless others. Under such harrowing circumstances, fake news regarding the possibility of the virus being a weapon of biological warfare, and the leakage of the virus from a lab working on genetic manipulations within viruses, did the rounds and scared people unnecessarily. The possibility of lab manipulation and the subsequent leak caused anger among people who lost a tremendous deal owing to the virus. However, consistent research and analysis into the virus' origin has helped discern the fact that, indeed, the novel coronavirus is not a product of human manipulation but rather the result of natural selection.

One of the major studies disproving the manipulation theory was conducted by Professor Long Liu of the Hubei University of Medicine. Under the well-documented study, the professor, along with his expert colleagues, studied multiple variants of SARS-CoV-2 occurring in different mammal species. The viruses thus isolated were then compared to the initial "Wuhan" circulating strain of the virus captured within the first wave of the pandemic. It is notable that, during subsequent waves, the virus mutated significantly, resulting in additional panic and the need for greater effort in devising a vaccine which may be effective against all possible variants. The Hubei University team of scientists used SARS-CoV-2 genome sequences collected from mammals including humans, cats, dogs, tigers, lions, ferrets and mink. Following the collation of the virus genomes, the sequences were utilised to construct a phylogenetic tree which would enable the researchers to understand the evolutionary history of the viruses. An adaptive evolution server named Datamonkey was then leveraged to identify branches which indicated that the virus had been under selective pressure. The next step involved Liu and colleagues using the codon adaptive index to study the variety of mutations visible in the different virus variants.

The outcome of the detailed study, which formed the basis of several subsequent studies, indicated that the novel coronavirus binds to the ACE-2 enzymes frequently located outside respiratory cells and the virus, by way of this binding, then accesses and infects the human cell. The study indicated, as depicted earlier, that the virus originated from zoonotic sources and not lab manipulation. The host could either be bats or pangolins, there is no conclusive proof of the same as of yet. However, there is adequate proof to conclusively state that the lab theory around the origin of the novel coronavirus, which created panic and anxiety among the global population, is absolutely bogus and of no scientific relevance.

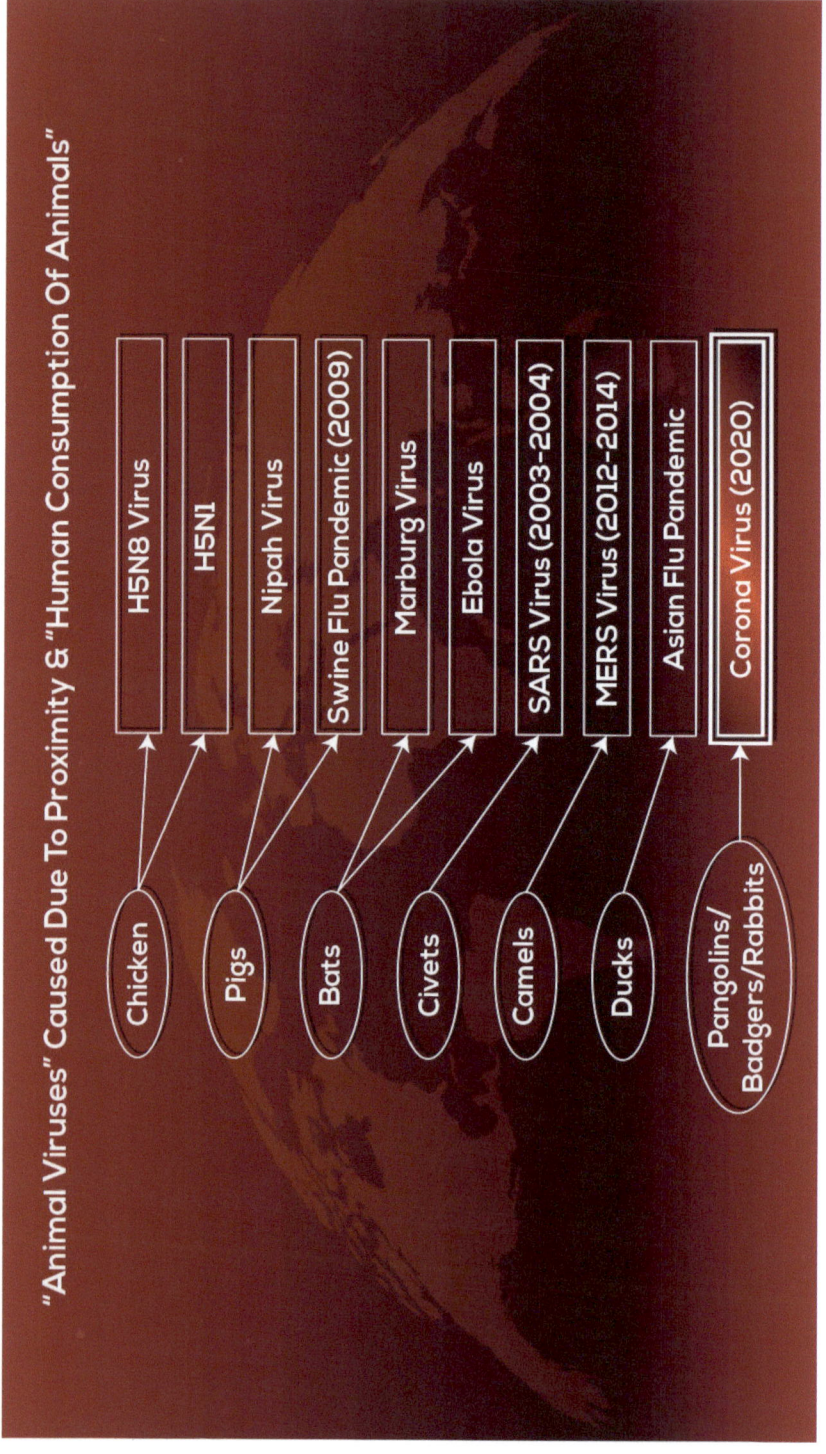

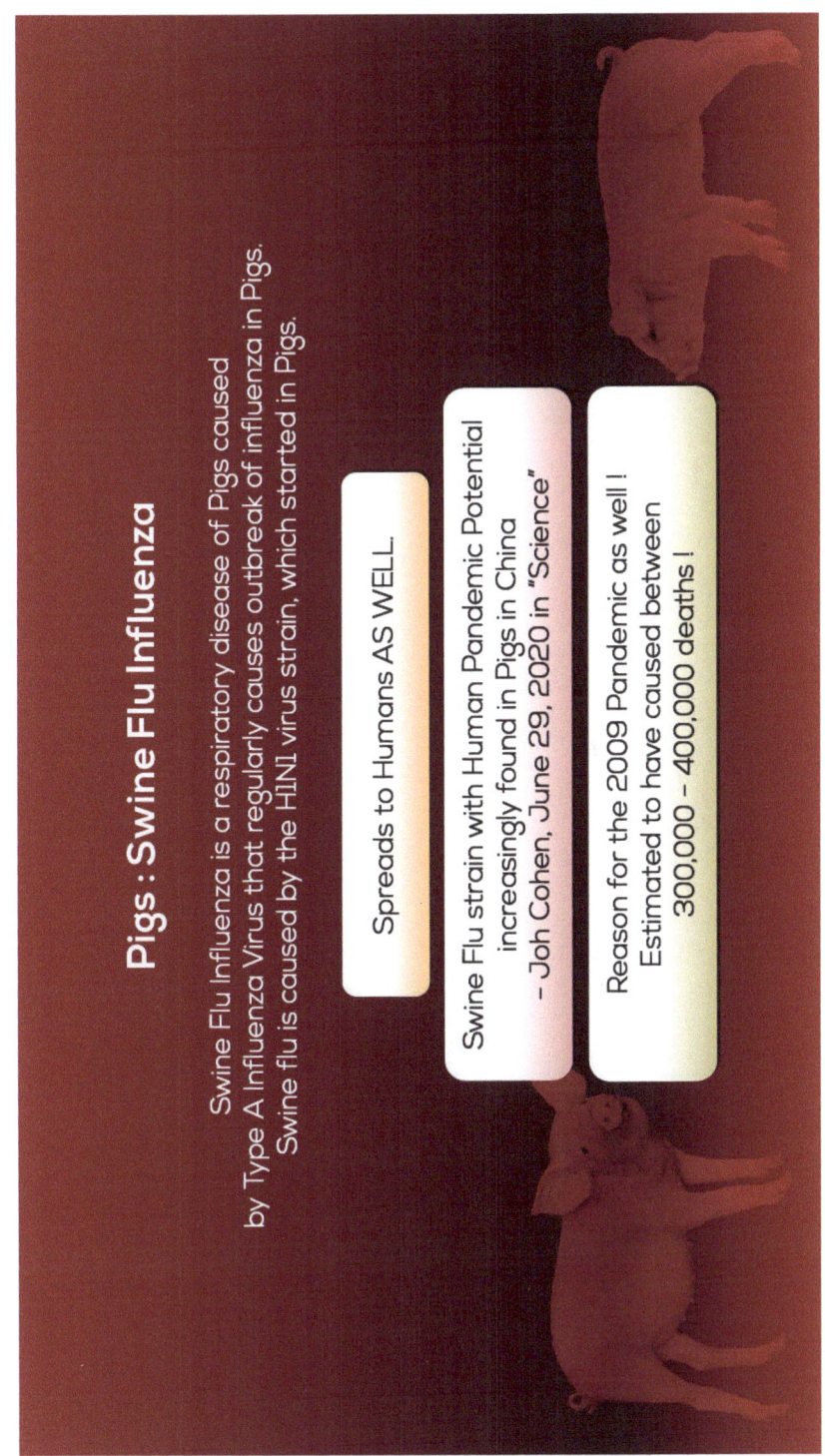

"US Livestock Meat Packing Plants Contributes 6-8% of US Covid 19 Cases"

- "New research published by the National academy of series ties livestock meat packing plants to 6-8% of US Covid 19 case, and 3-4% of the deaths through late July".

- Authors shows that there is a "strong positive relationship" between meat packing plants + "local community transmission" suggesting the plants act as "transmission vectors" and "Accelerate the Spread of the Virus".

- Communities that acted to shut down slaughterhouses reduced spread, according to the researchers.

- Study estimated Meat packing Plants were associated with 236,780 to 310,000 Covid 19 cases and 4360 to 5250 deaths by July 21.

Study by Chicago Booth (University of Chicago) Columbia University School of Int'l 8 Public Affairs (2020). (Bloomberg, Mike Dorning, Nov 23 2020).

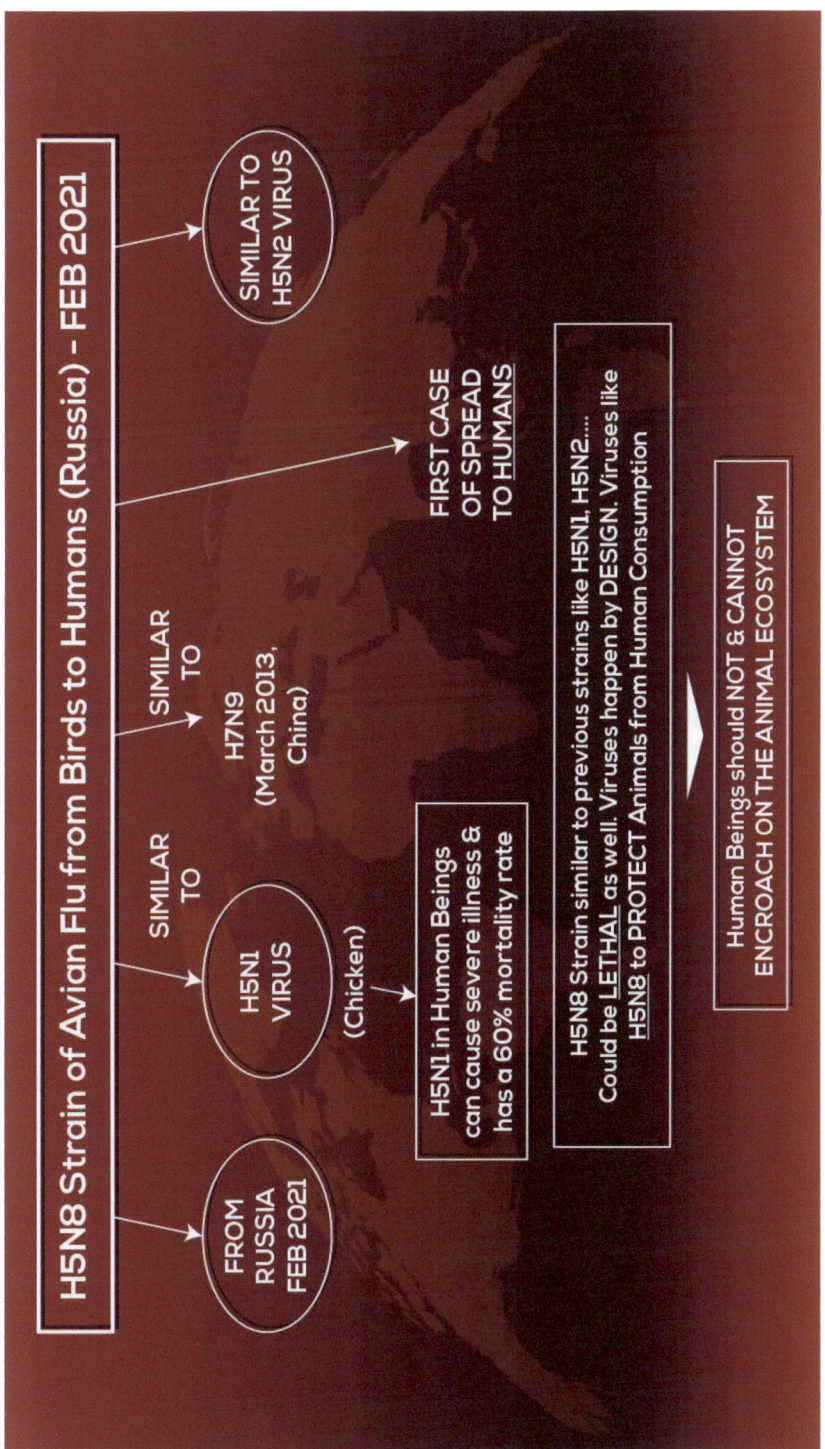

Human consumption of Civets : SARS virus

Jan 2004/cts : "Chinese authorities have ordered the deaths of some 10,000 Civets cats - a weasel like animal that is local delicacy and related wildlife by Saturday. Genetic tests have suggested a link between Civets and the SARS virus diagnosed in a 32 year old TV producer in Guangdong.

"WHO sees more evidence of Civet role in SARS"
by Robert Roos, Jan 16, 2004
(Center for Infectious Disease Research & Policy)

Robert Roos
Jan 16 2004

COVID 19: Why the Lab Theory is Bogus! | 75

Human consumption of Camels : MERS VIRUS

- MERS was caused due to consumption of camels in the MIDDLE EAST.
- MERS was "LOCALIZED", hence did NOT spread.
- In the case of COVID-19 (CORONA VIRUS), regular 4-6 flights/day from Wuhan to USA, Iran & Europe. The virus spreads. Birth of Pandemic.

> MERS due to human consumption of "Camels"
> MERS "LOCALIZED", hence did NOT spread.
> Corona spread due to 4-5 daily flights to USA, Europe & Iran

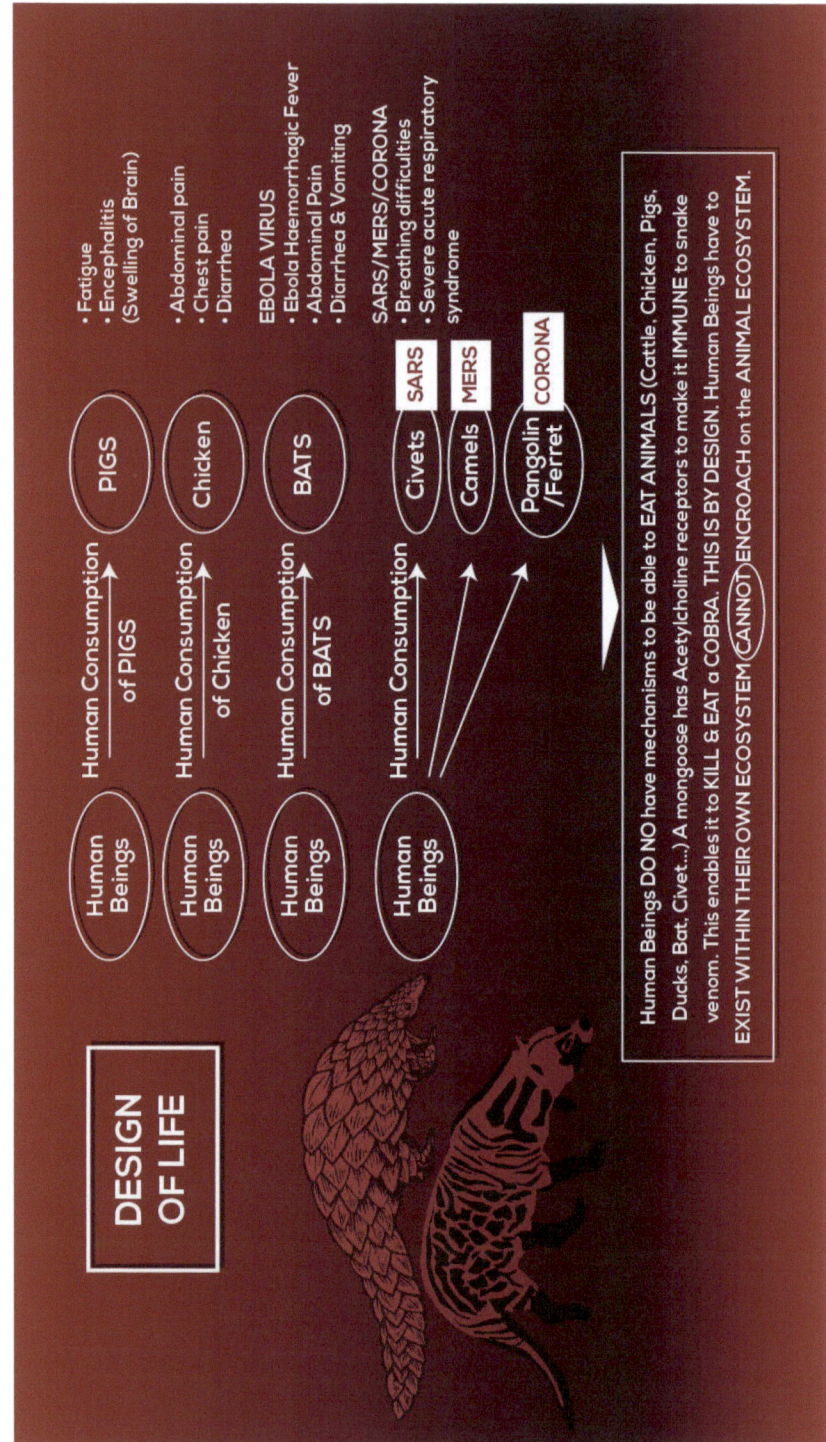

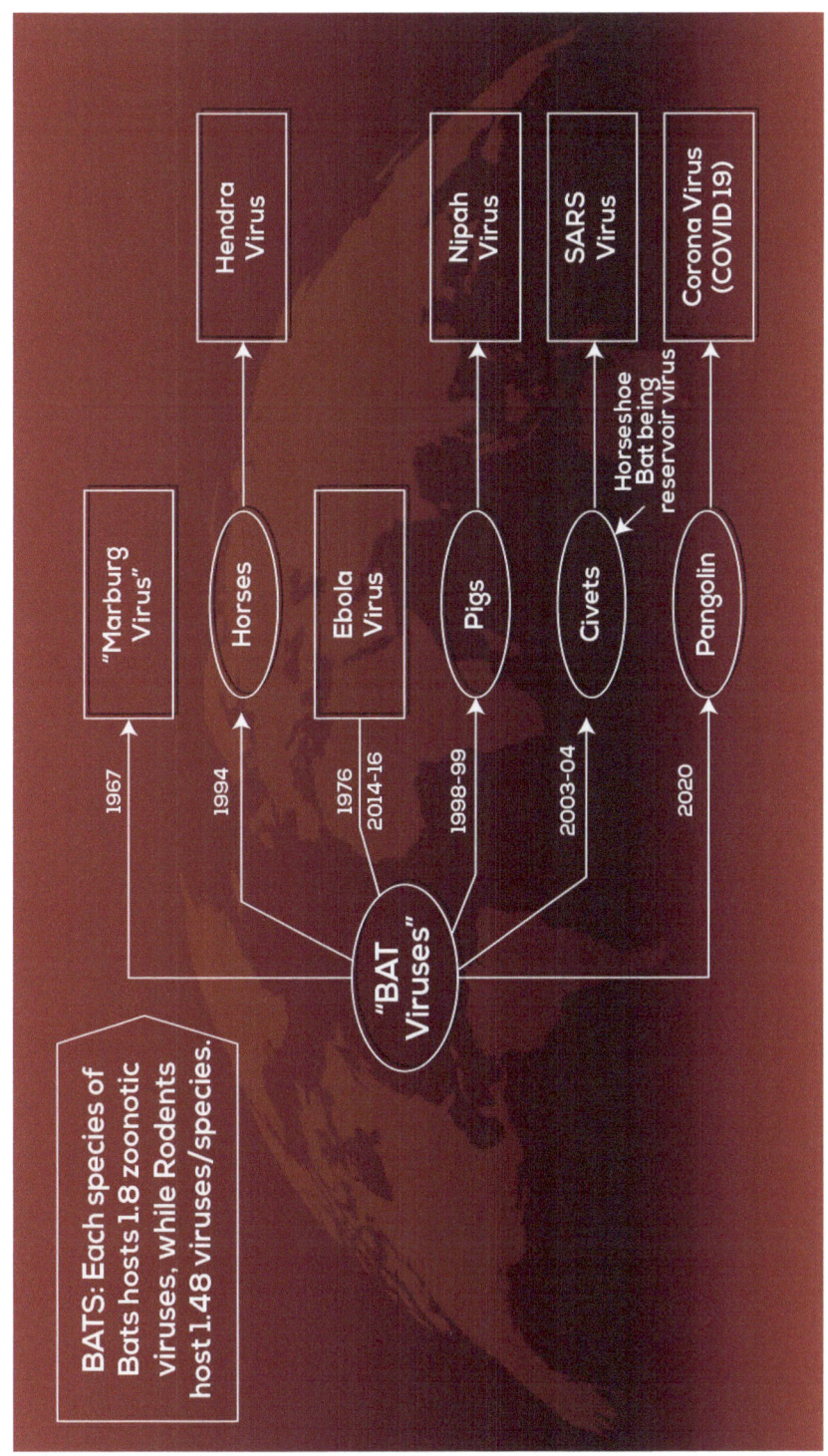

The Killer Bat

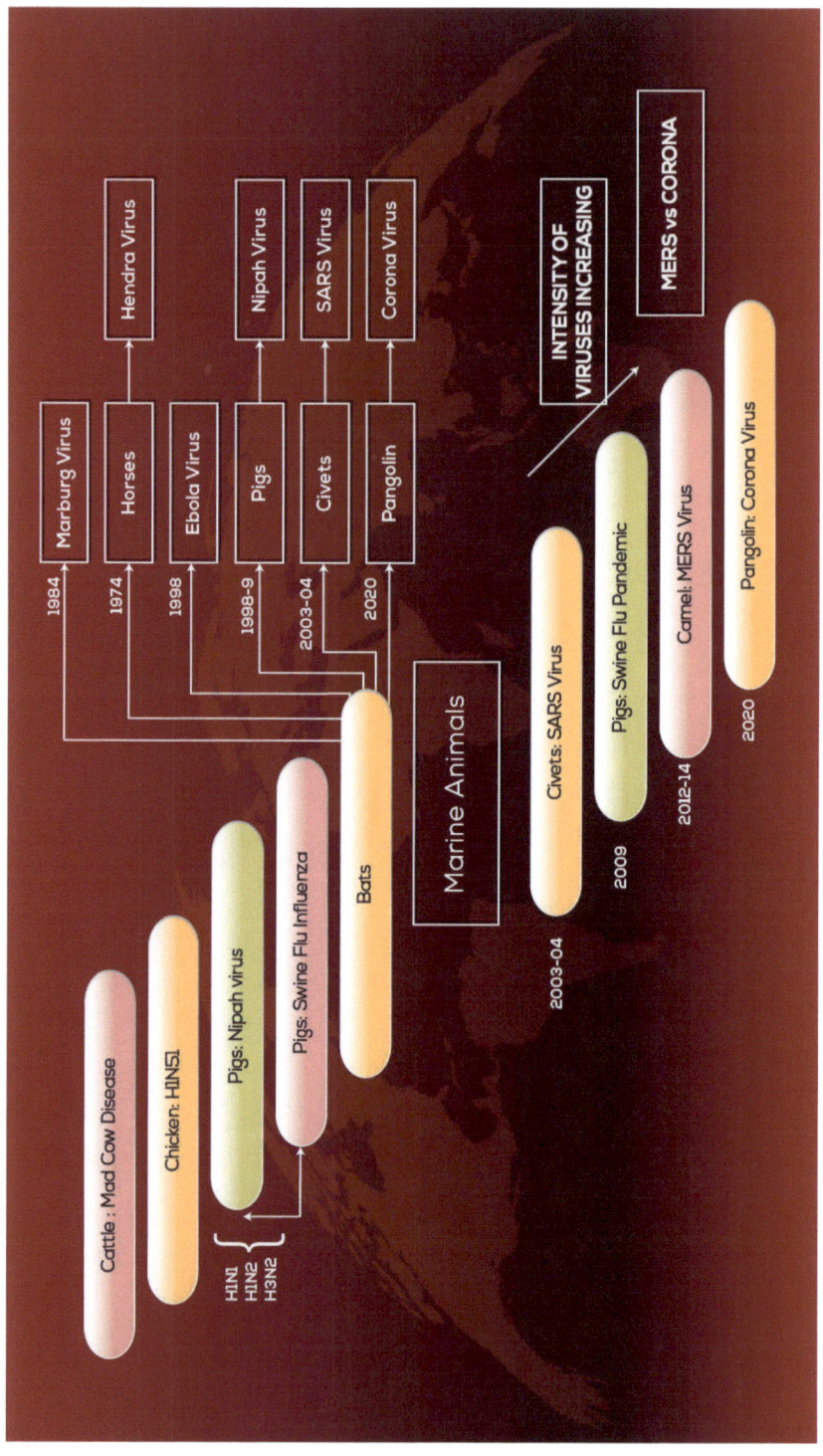

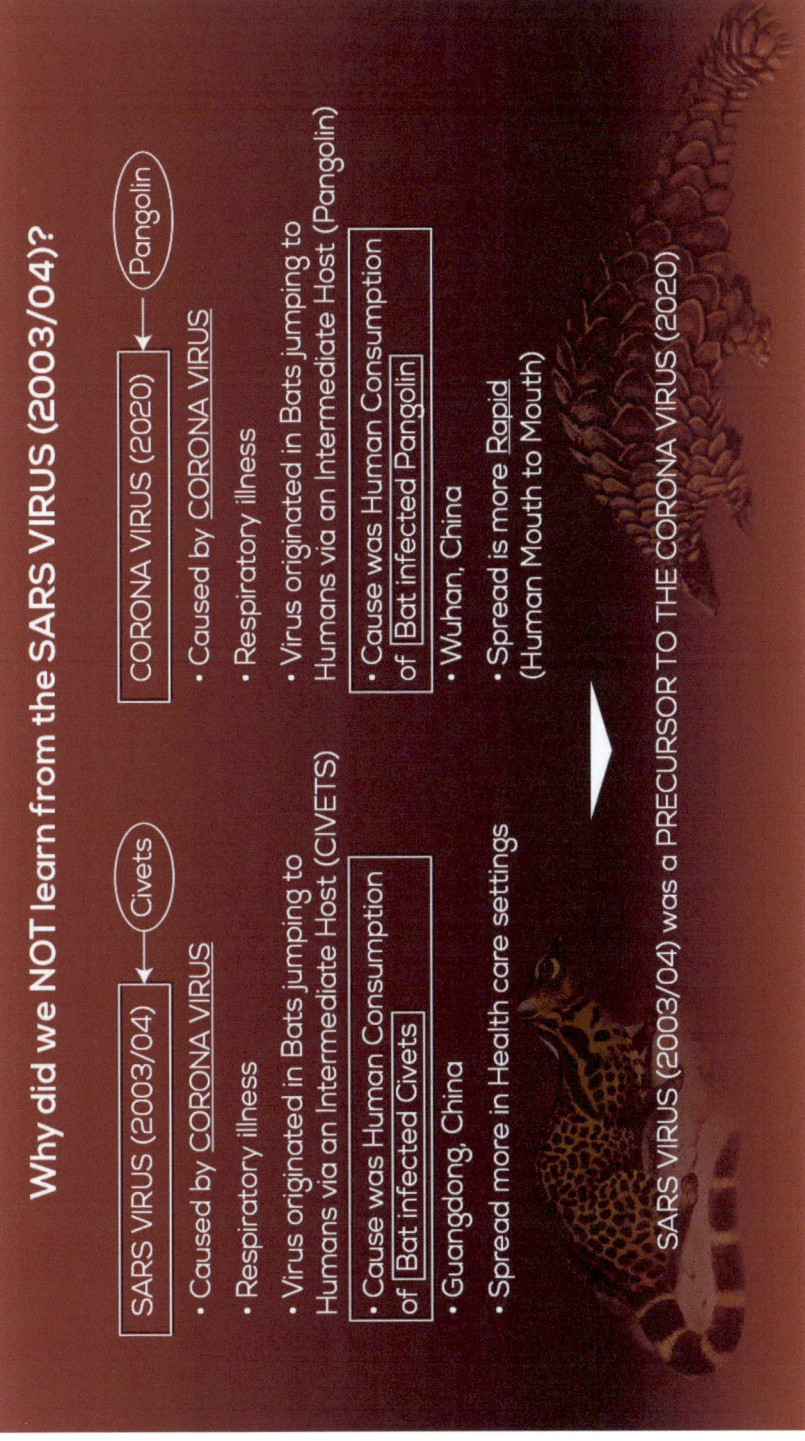

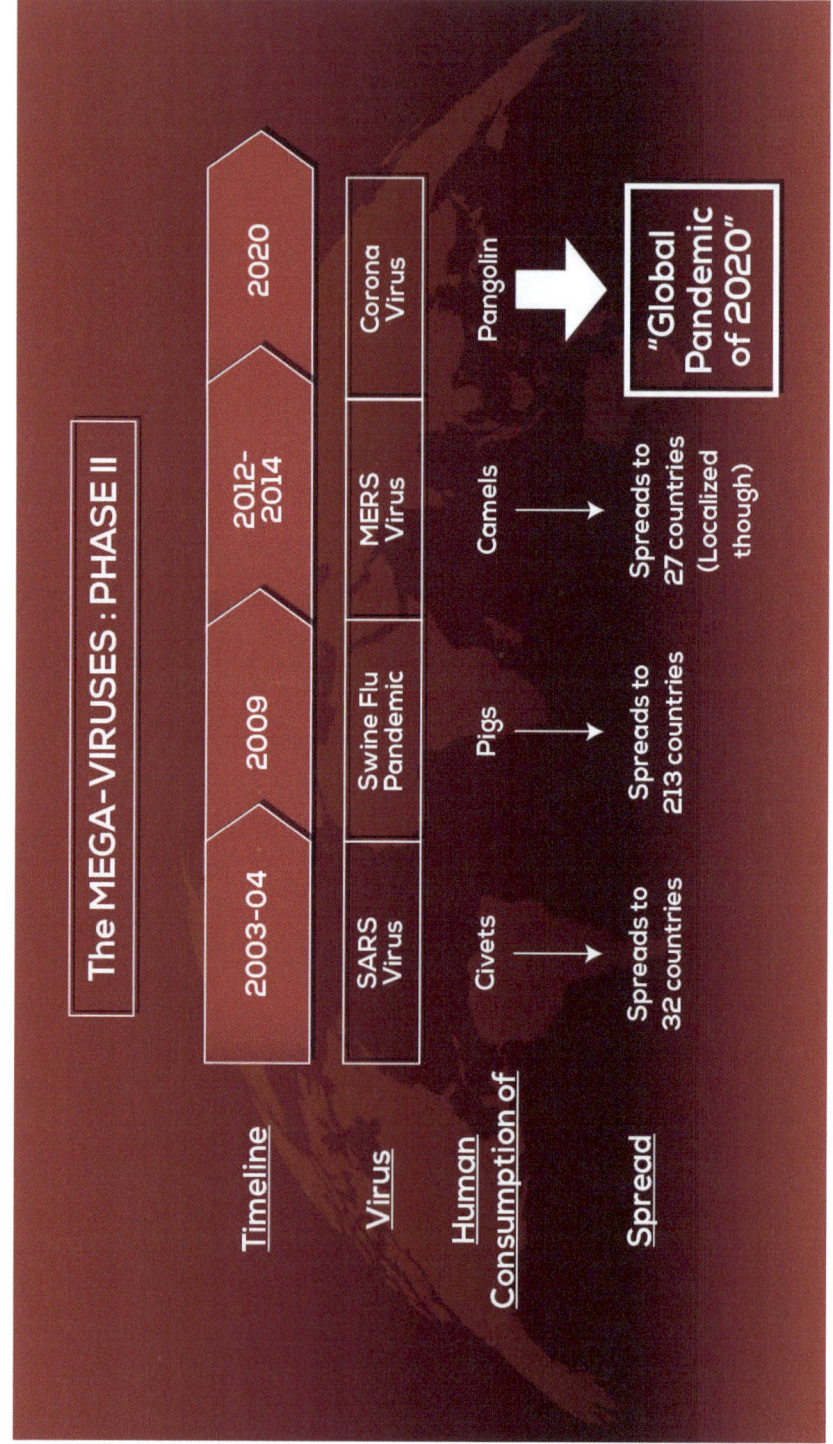

COVID 19: Why the Lab Theory is Bogus! | 81

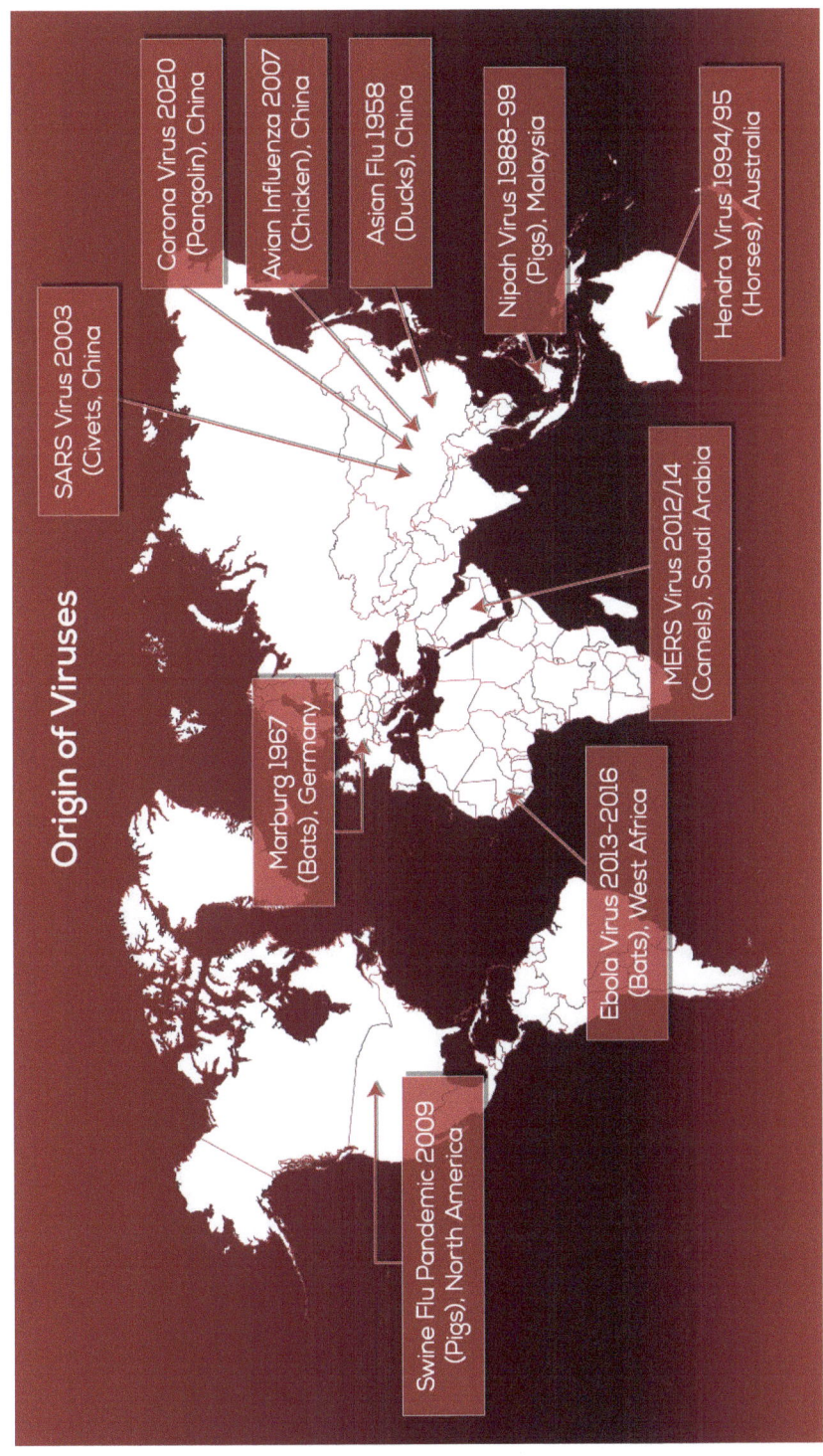

The Killer Bat

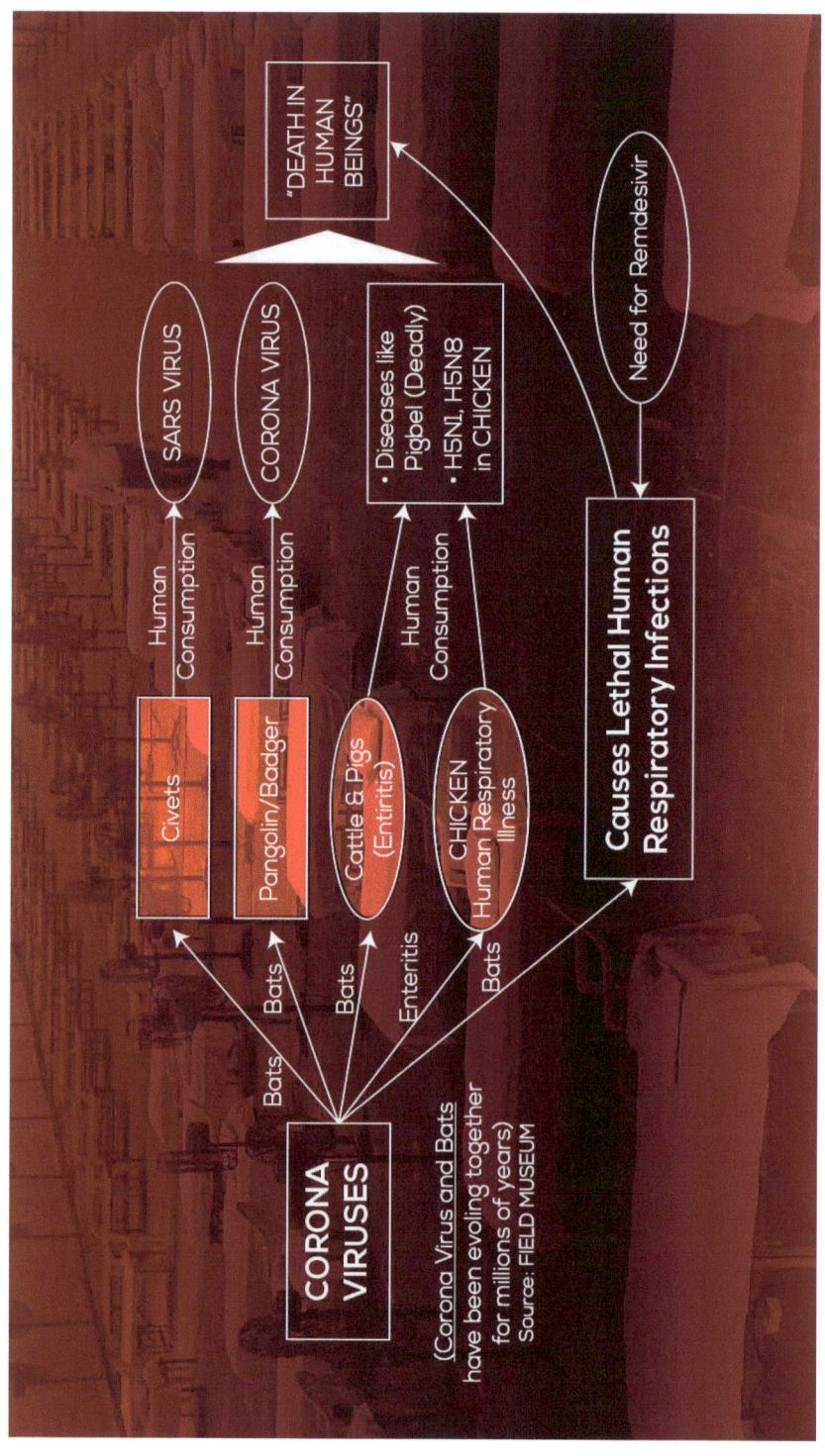

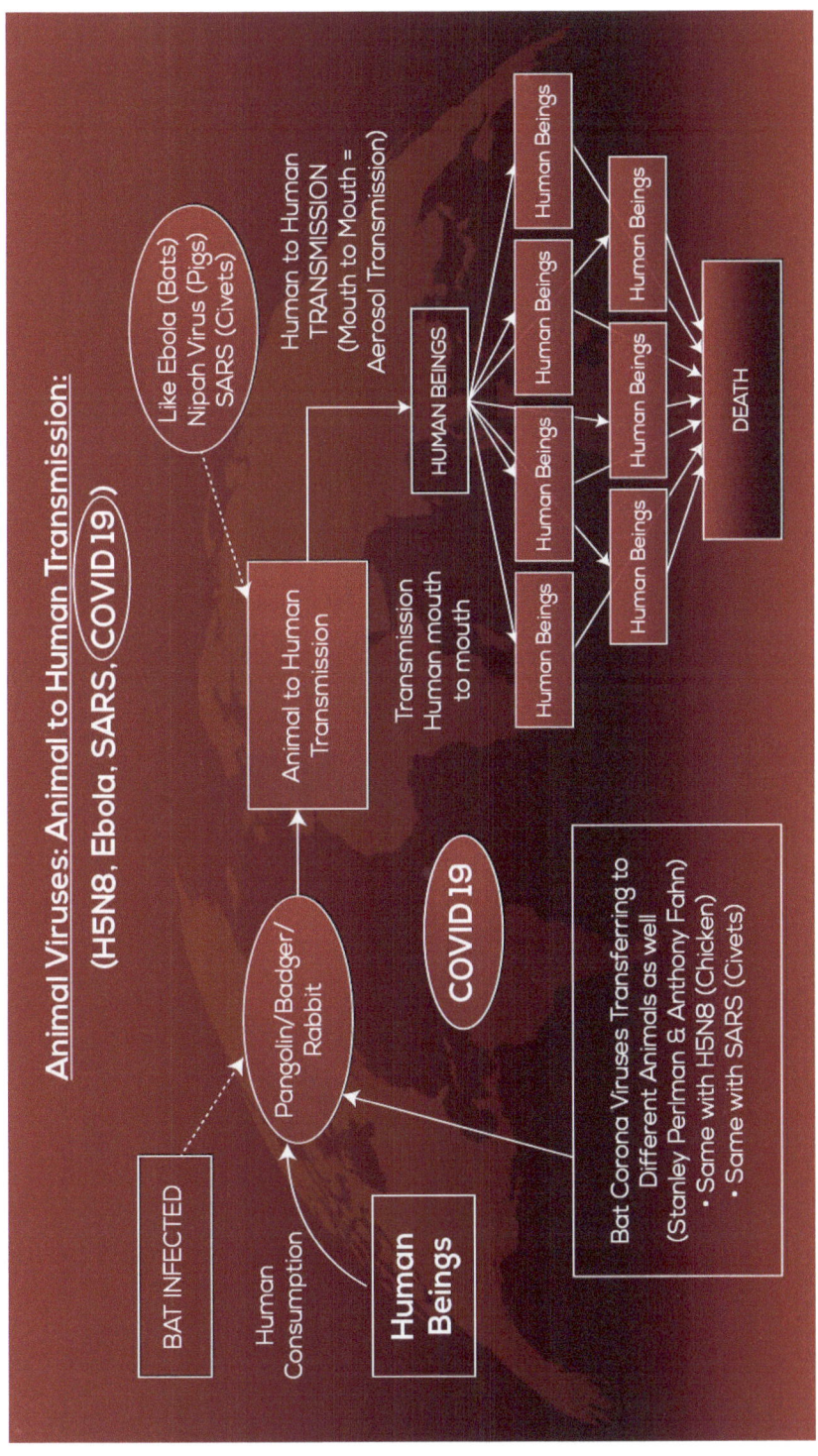

The Killer Bat

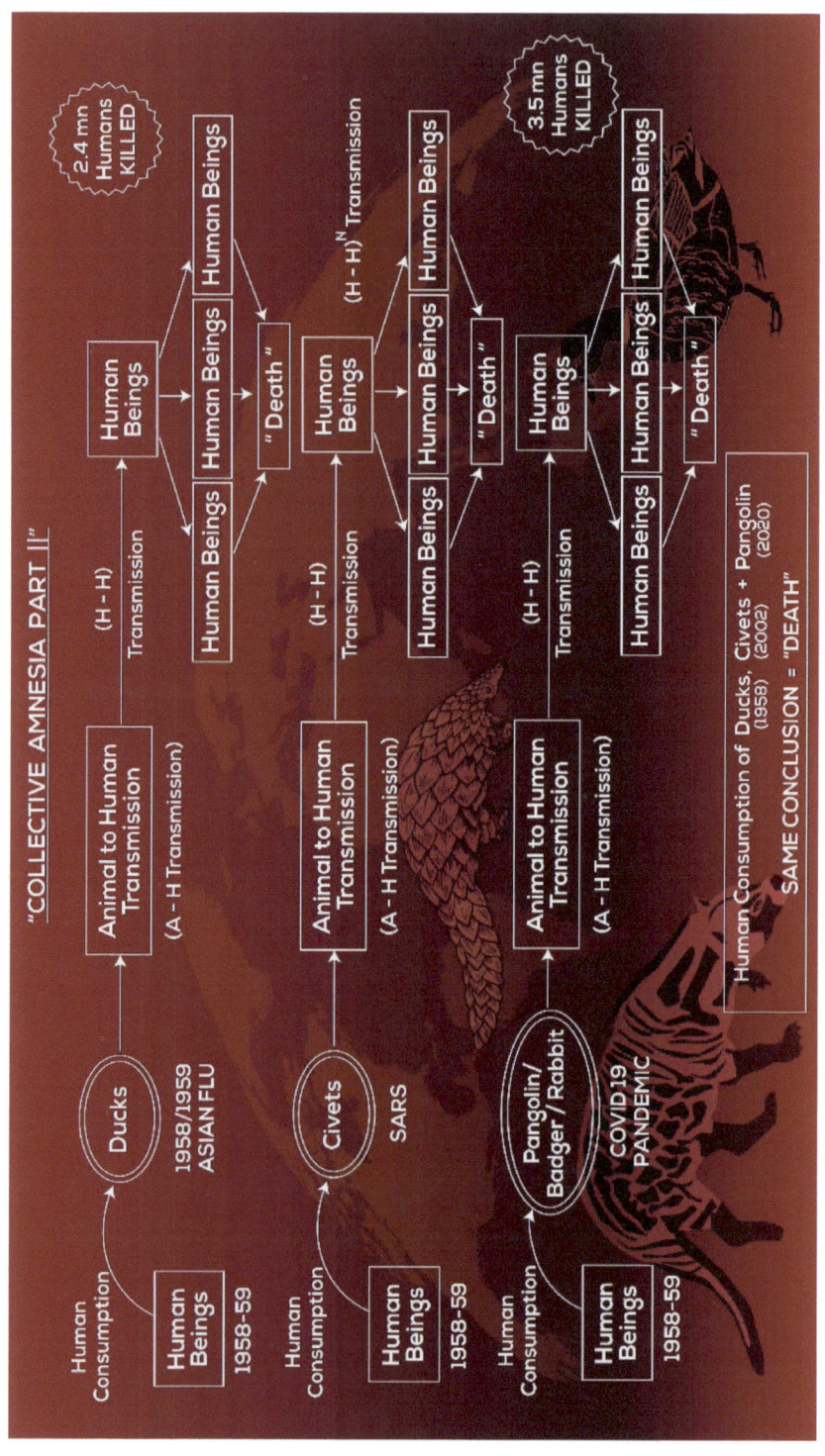

HUMAN BEINGS CANNOT ENCROACH ON THE ANIMAL ECOSYSTEM:

Human Beings are a separate ECOSYSTEM from the Animal Ecosystem

The Animals Ecosystem is a CLOSED Ecosystem. Cobra venom reacts differently with Human Beings as against with a Mongoose. This is by DESIGN.

Human Beings CANNOT ENCROACH on the Animal Ecosystem

Cannibals also CANNOT ENCROACH ON THE HUMAN ECOSYSTEM. THEY get BRAIN DISEASE if they do.

If Human Beings had learnt lessons from SARS & MERS, COVID 19 would NOT have happened! 2m Precious LIVES would HAVE BEEN SAVED.

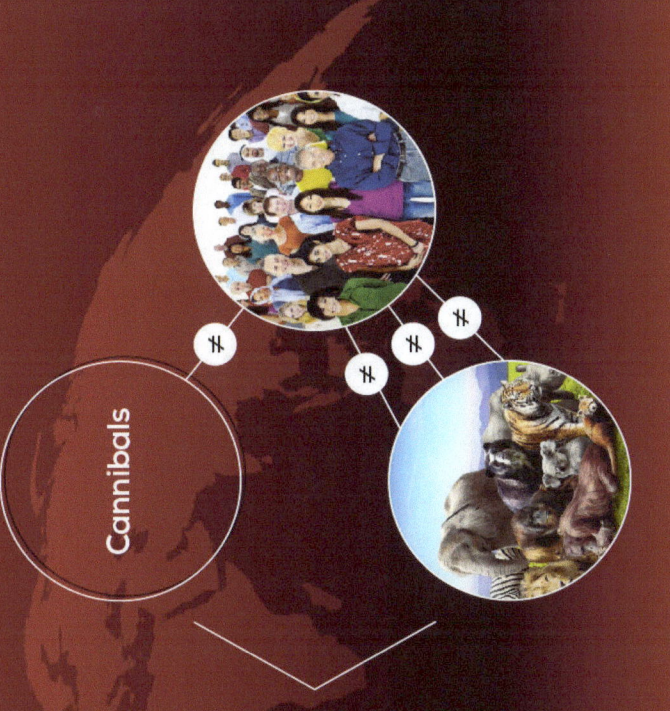

Cannibals

The Killer Bat

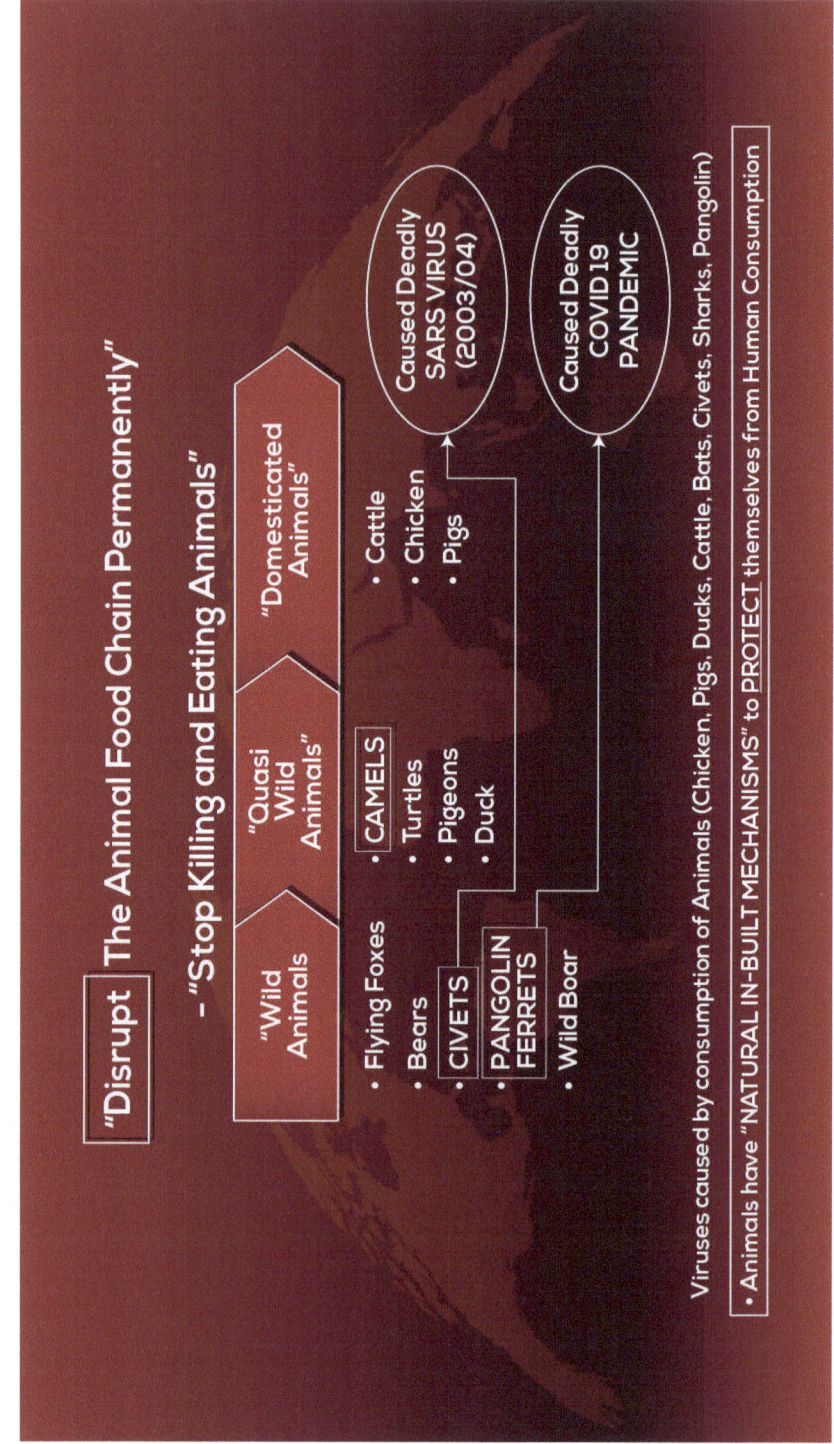

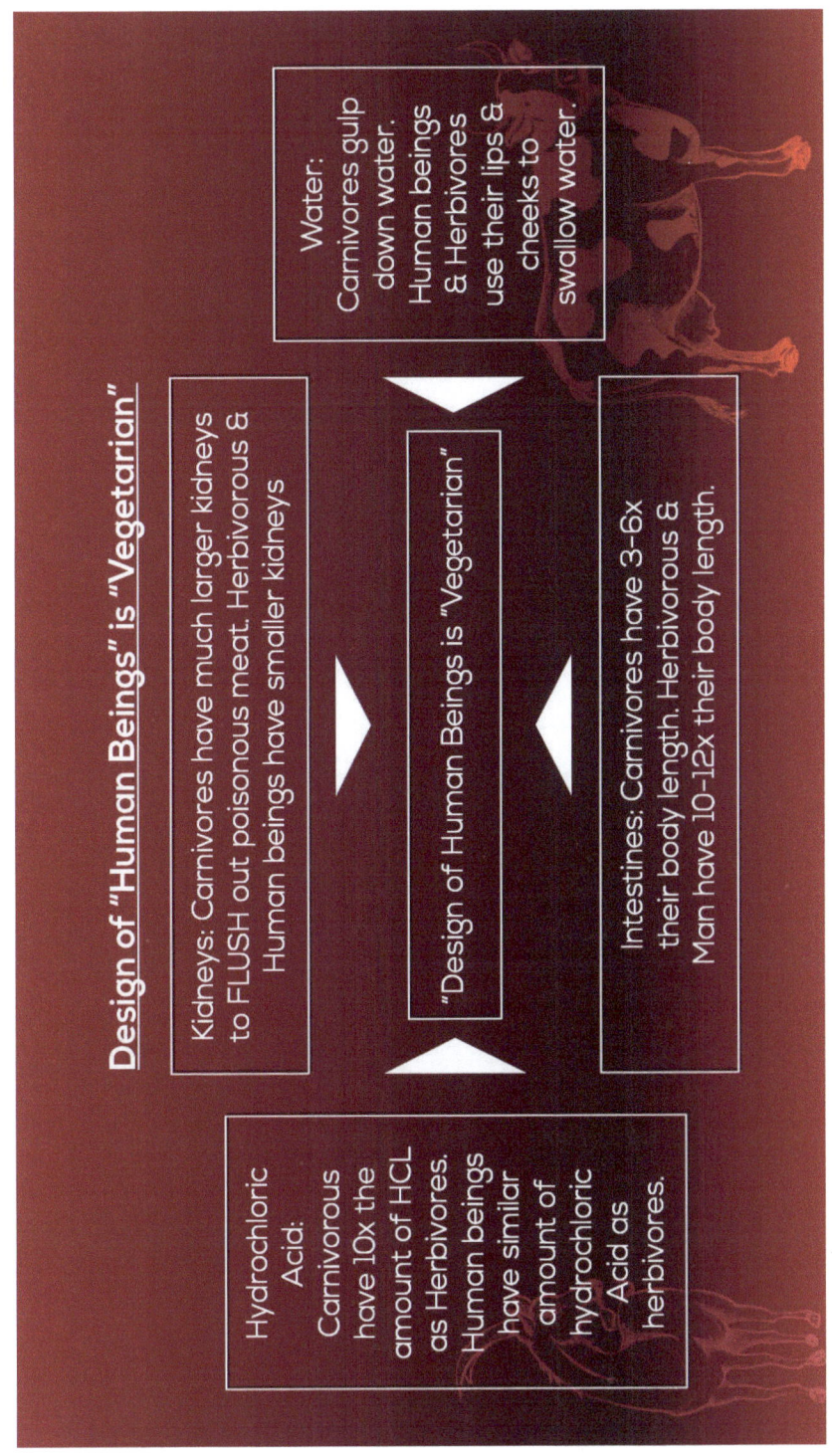

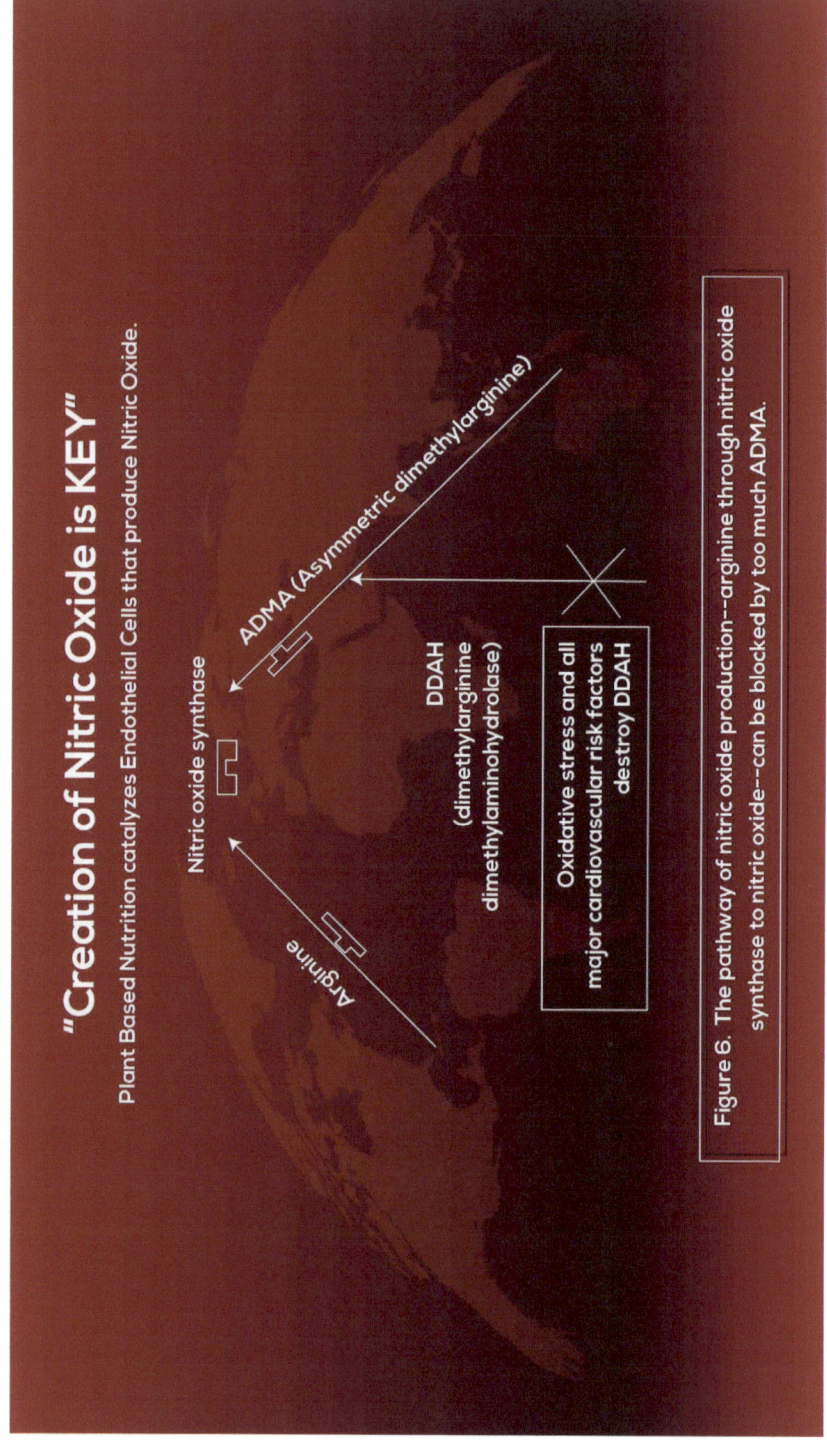

Figure 6. The pathway of nitric oxide production—arginine through nitric oxide synthase to nitric oxide—can be blocked by too much ADMA.

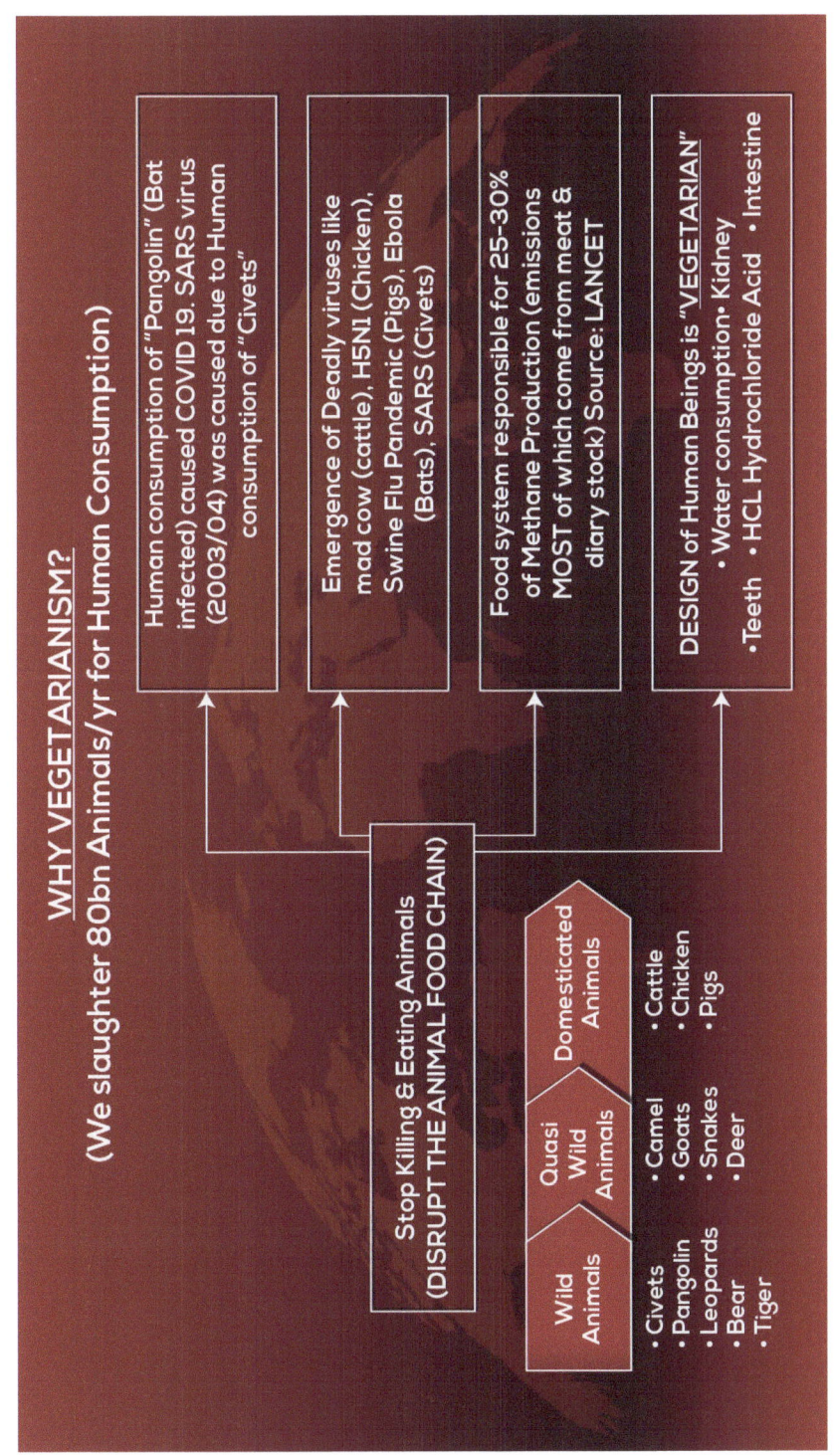

The Killer Bat

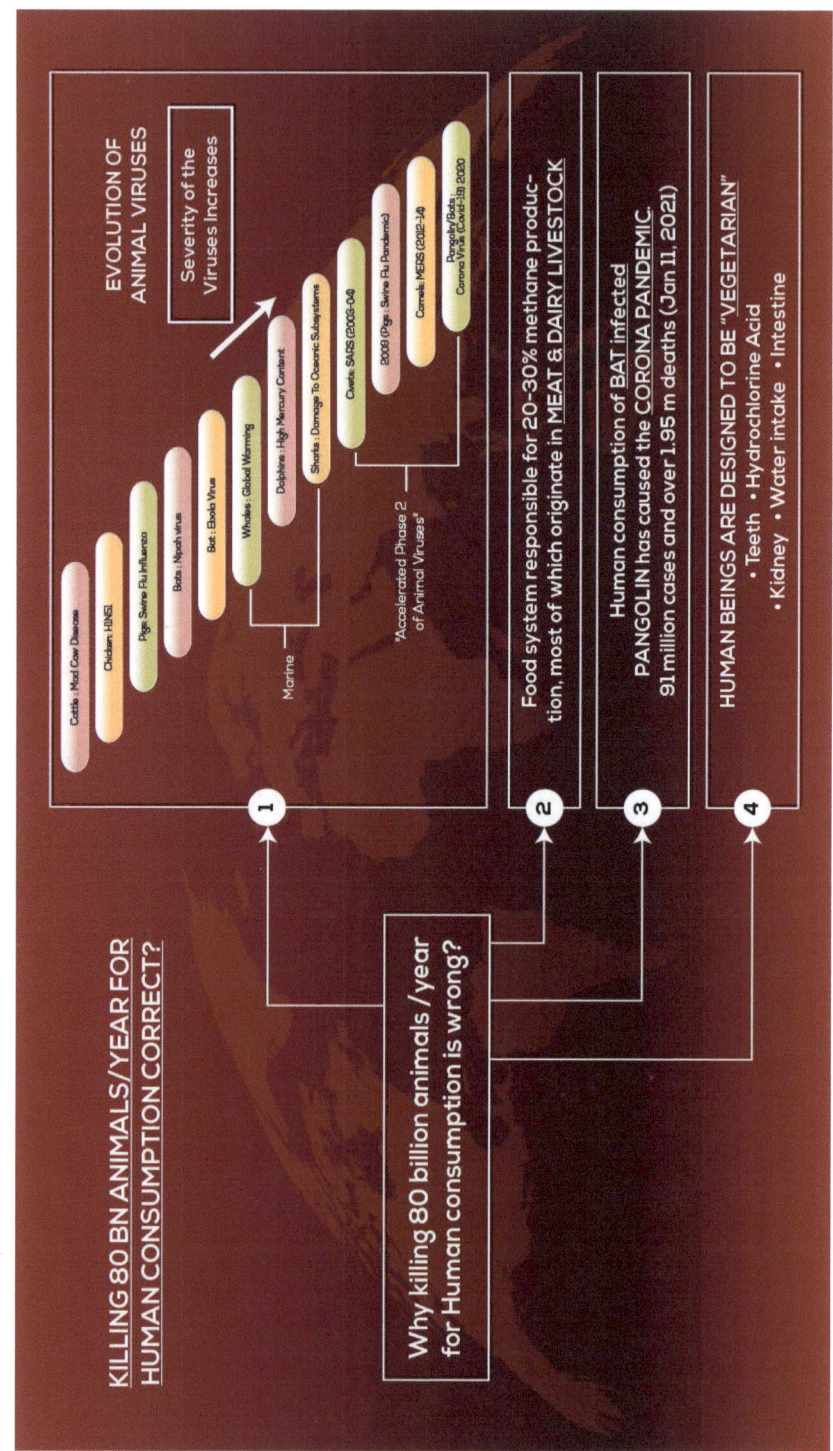<!-- Infographic: "KILLING 80 BN ANIMALS/YEAR FOR HUMAN CONSUMPTION CORRECT?" -->

COVID 19: Why the Lab Theory is Bogus!

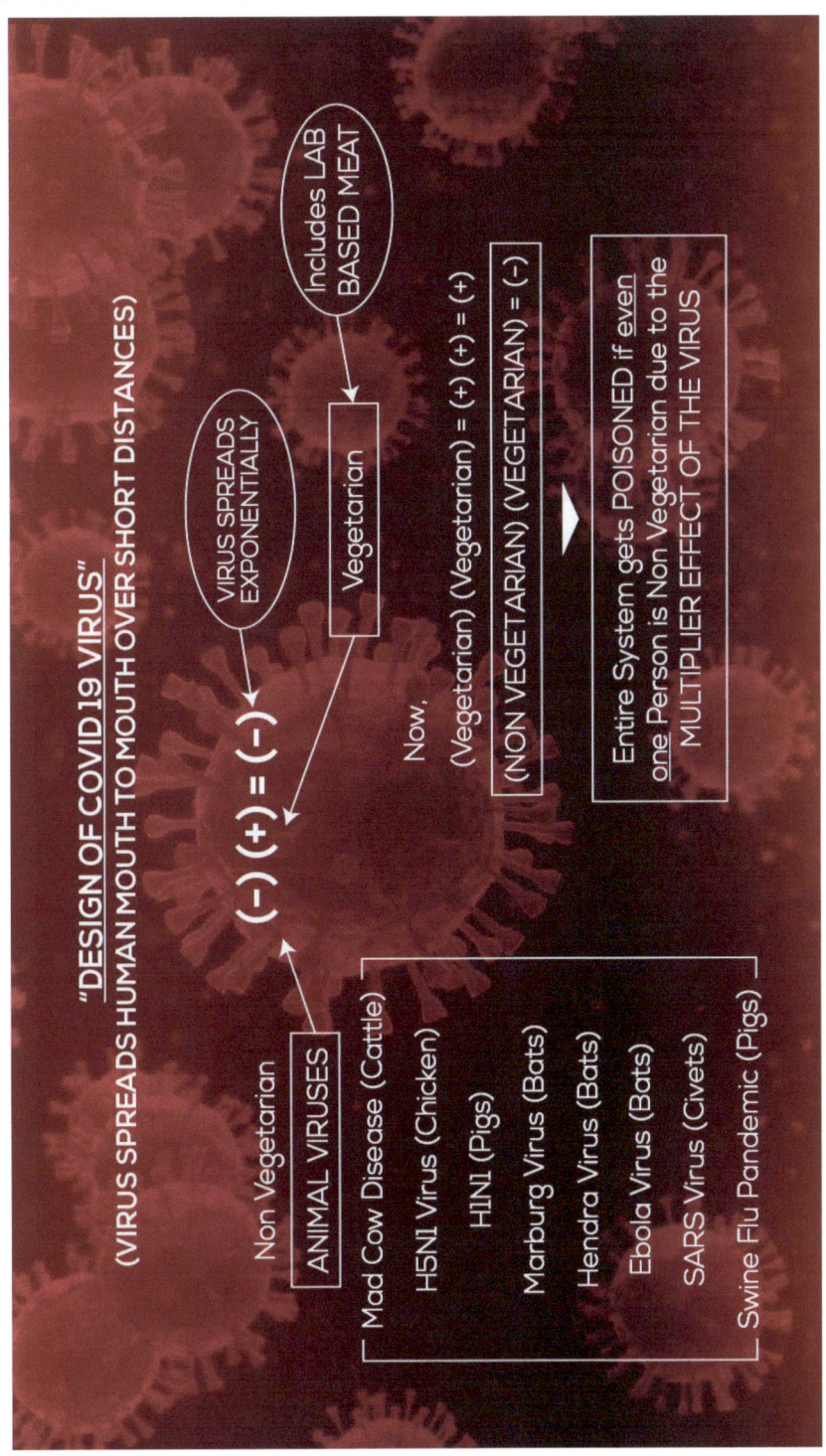

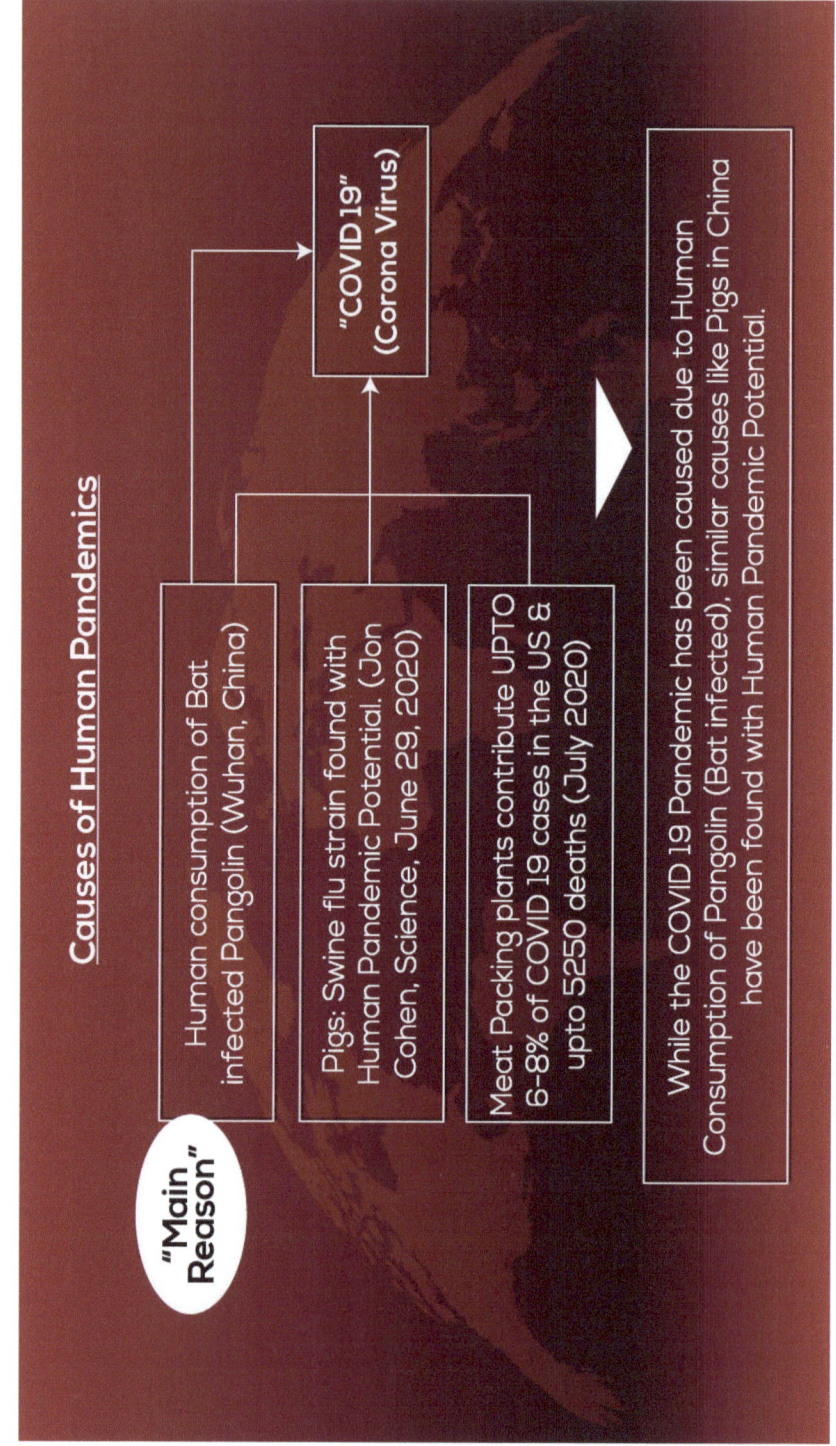

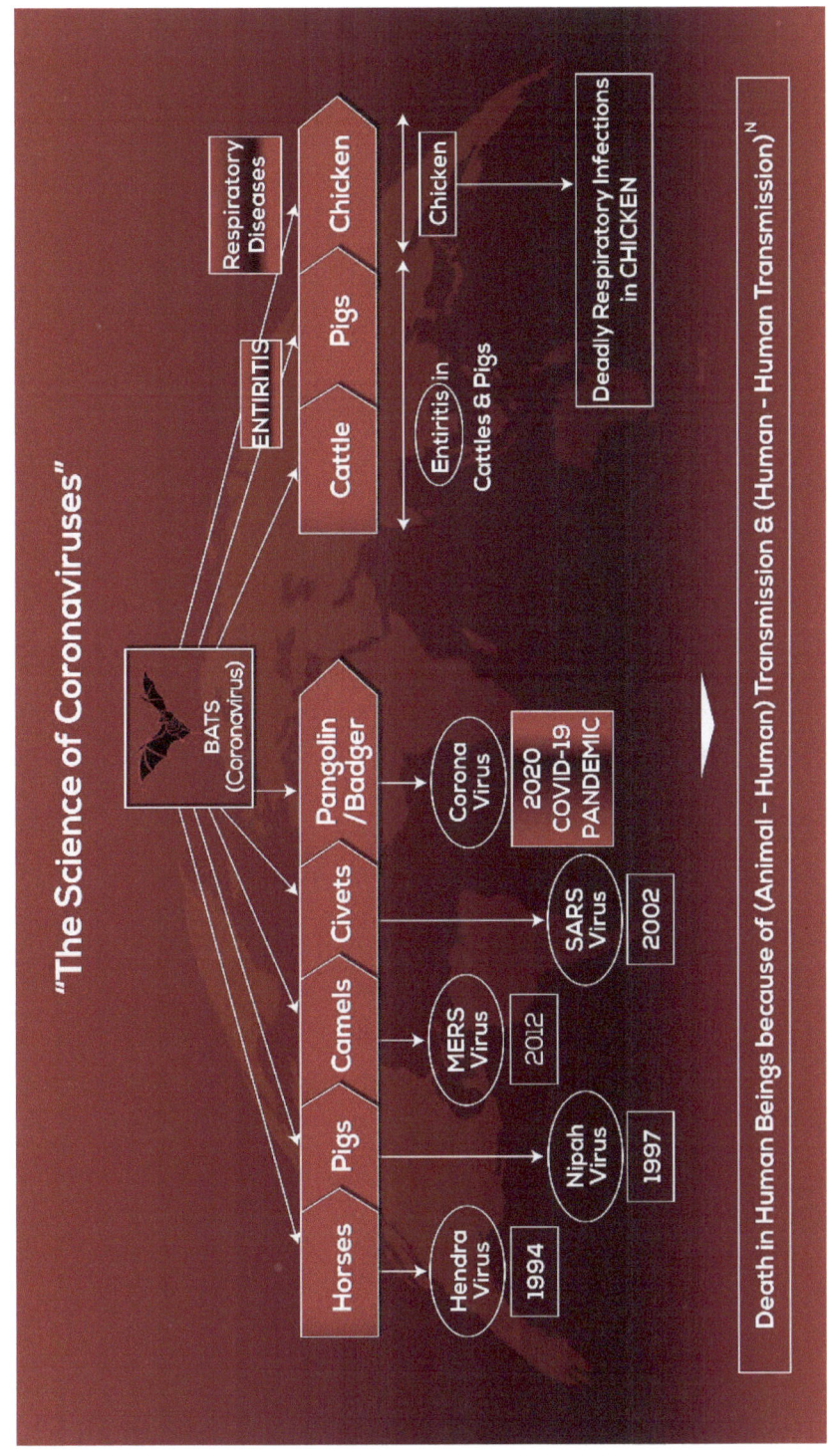

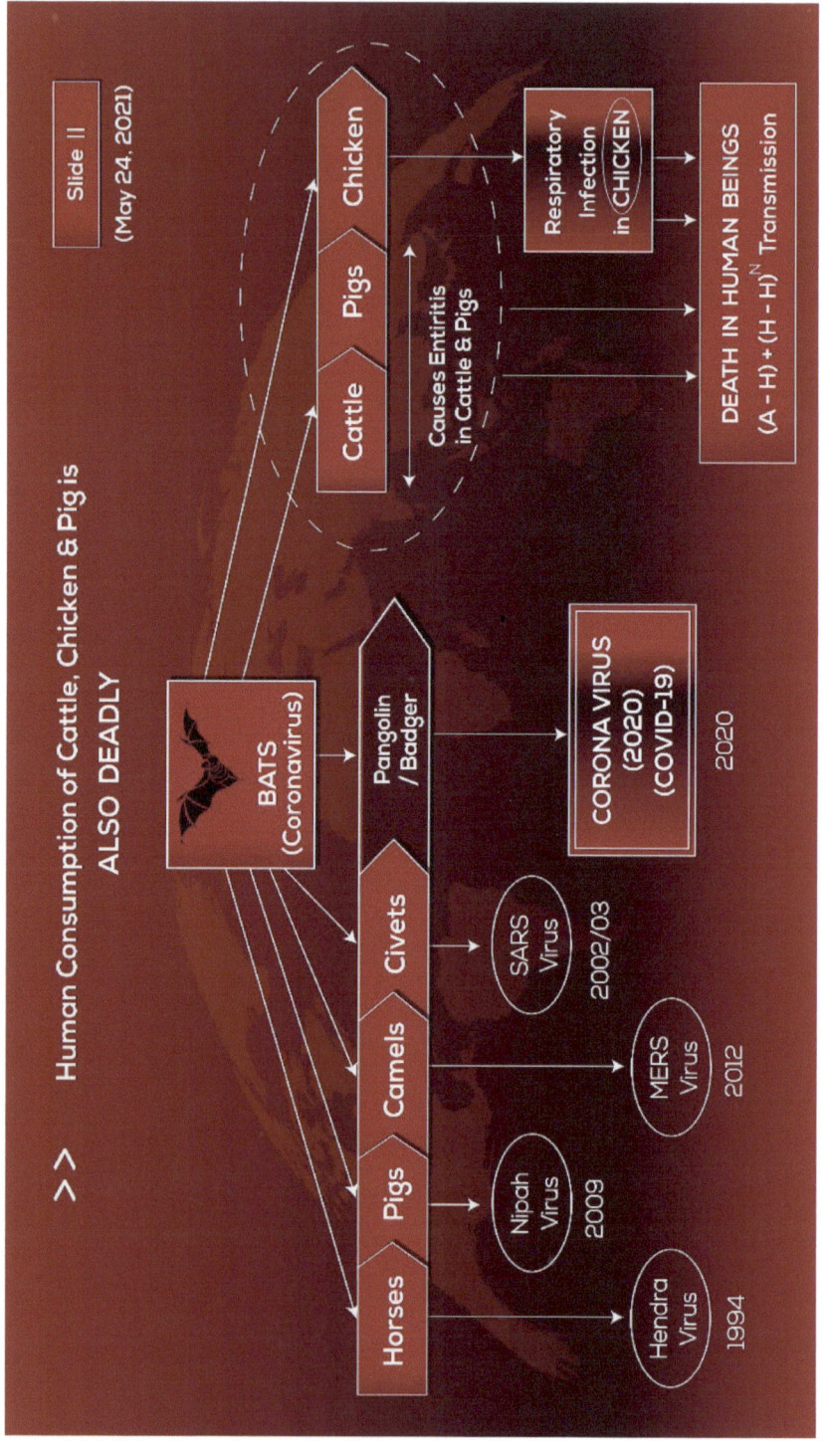

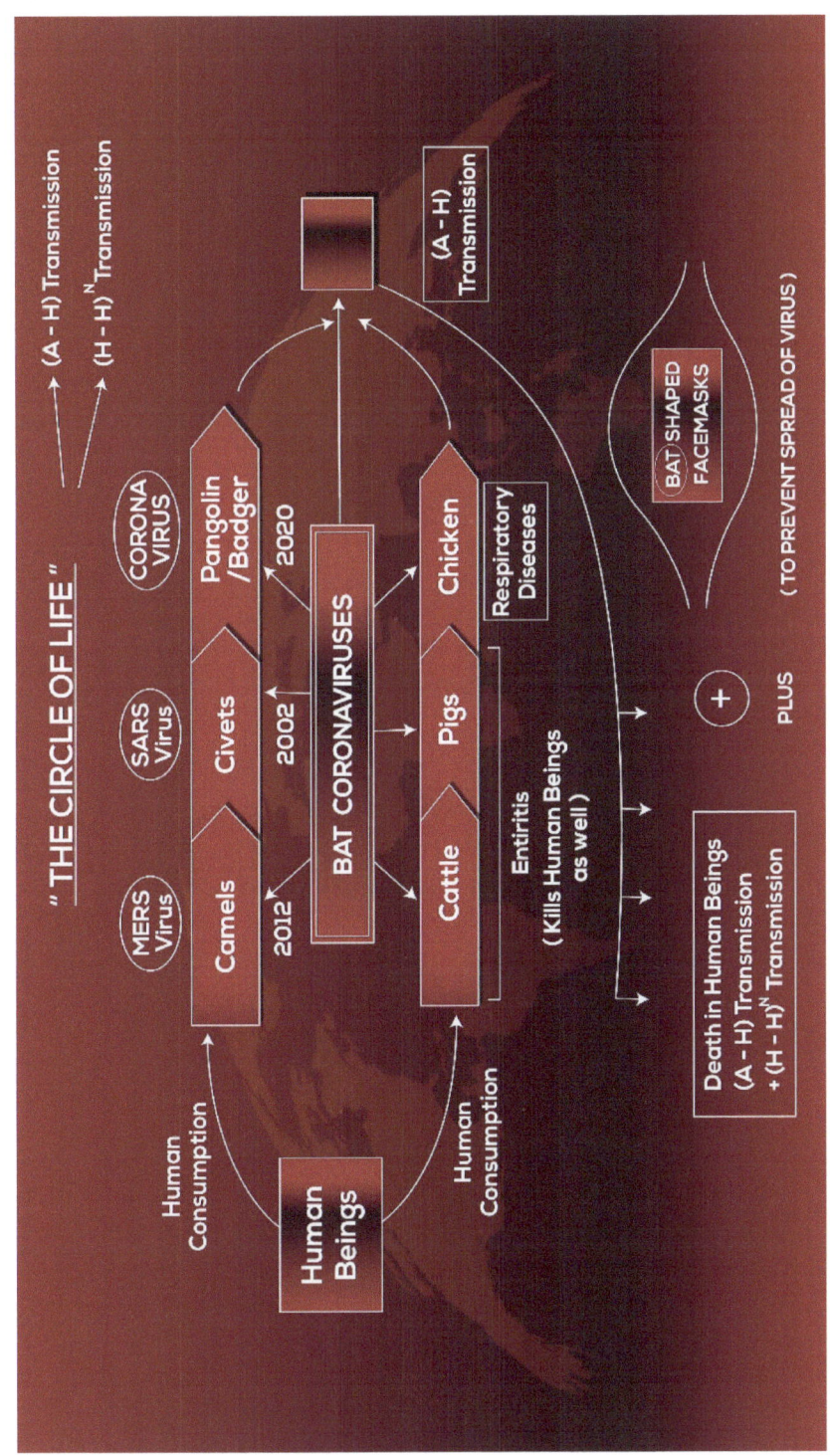

Chapter 7

Why Have Most of the Major Viruses Come from China?

Several studies indicate that a majority of the recent virus-led epidemics have had their origins in China, leading people to question why this is the case. As the world's most populous country, with a vibrant culture and historical background, China is one of the most exotic and interesting tourist destinations for global travellers. However, with the frequent virus outbreaks, people are beginning to worry about China's wellbeing. Indeed, China has emerged as the hotbed of new diseases, with a number of deadly viral infections stemming from the region.

Exhibit 12: Geographical origin of viruses

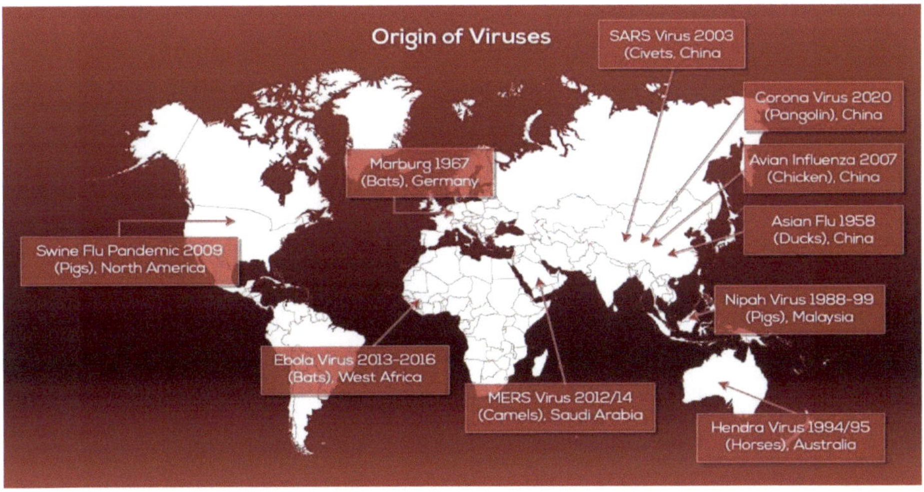

The ongoing global pandemic, caused by the novel coronavirus, or SARS-CoV-2, also originated in China and the contagion has already claimed an unprecedented number of lives and livelihoods across the globe. With multiple mutations and vaccine-resistant variants coming to the fore, the pandemic has wreaked havoc on a global scale and threatened the health and economic wellbeing of several countries. The fast-transmitting virus with a high infectious capability originated in the city of Wuhan in China towards the end of 2019, and has now spread to almost all countries across the globe.

Several investigations have taken place into the virus, which has forced the world to go into mandatory lockdowns and social distancing measures as a safeguard against the illness. While scientists are still debating over whether the zoonotic virus reached humans through bats or pangolins, there is concurrence over the possibility of the virus originating from the sale of live animals in the enormous live produce market in Wuhan. Previously, the 2003 SARS outbreak was also linked to the animal market in China and the H7N9 outbreak of 2013 was linked to the sale of live birds in the country. Studies have stated that China is privy to a number of unsafe human-animal interactions, leading to the spread of most zoonotic viruses which are transferred from these animals to humans and then further transmitted to other human beings, resulting in a nation-wide or global pandemic as seen currently. The biggest factor here is the fact that most wet markets in China house live animals in closed spaces, leading to quick transmission and mutation of dangerous viruses. Further, China's preference for fresh meat also creates multiple opportunities for human-animal interaction, leading to fatal infections and viral outbreaks.

7.1 Cultural and Historical Backdrop

China is a country of huge population and developed transport links, both major contributors towards the rapid spread of infectious diseases. Other than the recent SARS and H7N9 outbreaks, China has also been the land of origin of a new strain of coronavirus which infected and killed a number of piglets in 2016. However, the disease remained confined to the animals and did not spread to human beings.

While studying the various virus outbreaks in China, one of the major contentions is the cultural and historical background of the country.

The current Chinese culture is an amalgamation of old-world traditions and a westernized lifestyle based on the ethos promoted by the People's Republic. A unique co-existence of the two cultures is visible and can be termed as an example of the traditional Yin Yang formula of balance, exhibited by the intermingling of towering skyscrapers and heritage buildings. Boasting of a culture over 5000 years old, China's cultural history is varied and diverse. And the country's eating habits are an echo of this past steeped in tradition. One thing visible in recent China is the aspect wherein people are not as concerned with nutritional quality of food as the Western individuals. Rather, they are more focused on aspects such as the item's flavour, colour, aroma and texture, making them a nation of food enthusiasts and gastronomical adventurists.

Usually, Chinese meals include four major food classes – vegetables, grains, fruit, and meat. Most Chinese are lactose intolerant and prefer to stay away from dairy and dairy products. These are, therefore, substituted with large amounts of soymilk and tofu. However, the biggest contender in Chinese cuisine is meat, and people prefer their meat to be as fresh as possible. Some exceptions to the fresh meat rule include dried fish, beef jerky, and cuttlefish jerky but these are consumed much less voraciously than fresh meat. Furthermore, traditional Chinese cooking techniques do not favour deep frying or processing. People prefer their food raw or mildly cooked and only Western restaurants frequently serve deep fried food in China.

The affinity for freshly slaughtered meat is seen across the Chinese demographic, with people insisting that fresh poultry tastes much better and is healthier than refrigerated or frozen alternatives. And this is one of the major factors for the country being a hotbed for viral outbreaks. Put humans close to live produce markets with freshly slaughtered animals and there is a huge rise in the zoonotic transmission of viruses from animals to human hosts. Further, the sanitary situation in such live markets is also the cause for the origin of various life-threatening viruses.

There is another worrisome factor which might be a trigger for viral outbreaks in China – studies indicate that many Chinese residents prefer reaching out to traditional Chinese medicine practitioners, rather than Western medicine doctors, in the event of an illness. It is a sad state of affairs wherein these traditional practitioners misjudge the cause of the illness and prescribe medicines which do not help with the infection, leading to wide-spread transmission between humans. Such practices increase death rates and lead to the outbreak of a nation-wide, and subsequently, global pandemic affecting scores of lives and livelihoods. In the case of the ongoing pandemic itself, Chinese traditional medicine practitioners have prescribed an unproven liquid concoction consisting of Chinese skullcap, honeysuckle, and weeping forsythia, and the medicine is not known to alleviate the symptoms or the infection.

Another factor responsible for making the country a hotbed of viral outbreaks is the fact that China is infamous for its political policies involving misinformation, secrecy and state-level censorship which prevents residents from taking stock of their physical wellbeing. Such aspects prevent people from gaining important and adequate information, making them susceptible to widespread infection and subsequent death.

7.2 Theory of Animal Consumption

China is, undoubtedly, a country of meat lovers and people love their meat to be freshly slaughtered. This, in addition to the unhygienic conditions of the live produce markets, is a breeding ground for potential and previous virus outbreaks. It is a proven fact that the Chinese populace hardly waste any part of the animal. It is astonishing how they have found ways of cooking and consuming almost all portions of animals. Chinese residents are also known for their proclivity for a variety of meat, including animals and birds which may not be usually consumed by other people.

Reports state that the Chinese culture and tradition believes in "yi xing bu xing," a theory which says that consuming any part of the animal body strengthens and replenishes the same body part in human beings. Given such a belief when it comes to animal consumption, it is no surprise that Chinese residents prepare and eat almost all parts of animals.

An instance of the belief can be seen in the fact that Chinese consume shark fin soup and bird saliva as a means to strengthen the body and increase appetite while wisdom can be gained through the consumption of monkey's brains. Such food items are widely used as delicacies and tonics and usually served during special occasions and gatherings in China. While the theory adds colour and flavour to Chinese cuisine and culture, it also acts as a predecessor to viral outbreaks and subsequent global pandemics.

7.3 Recent Rise in Animal Consumption

China is a land of huge economic activity and development, and the rise of the middle class has led to a major increase in meat consumption across the country. Meat products have now become a major component of the Chinese meals and food sector and the country has a long and colourful tradition of livestock production and consumption of meat including poultry, lamb, beef and pork, along with more exotic items like bats and frogs. Once considered a luxury, meat has now transitioned into a staple diet for Chinese residents.

According to Statista, the country is now the world's biggest producer, consumer and importer of meat, and pork is the dominant meat in the market. Figures from 2018 suggest that the residents in China consumed over 41 kilograms of pork, per capita. In second and third place come poultry and beef. In an indication of the country's proclivity for meat, China's population currently consumes about 28% of the global meat supply.

While a large quantity of meat is produced within the country's borders, China also imports a substantial range and quantity of meat from foreign markets. 2019 saw the country increasing its meat import volume and diversifying its sources by importing meat from 16 new countries.

Going ahead, China's meat consumption is only set to increase, with production and consumption of less preferred meat items such as beef and lamb expected to rise at least 25% over the next ten years. According to Statista surveys, meat production volume in China stands at 77.5 million metric tonnes and the revenue of the meat produce market in China is recorded at 82.1 billion dollars.

Given the country's affinity for meat, and other factors discussed above, there is hardly any surprise over why China is a hotbed for viral outbreaks. Taking stock of the last century, epidemics including the flu contagion of 1918, 1957 and coronavirus outbreaks of 2002 and 2019 are attributed to China. Following the number of viral outbreaks, and the unprecedented scale of the ongoing contagion, people in China, and across the globe, are now expressing concern over the uncontrolled consumption of wild animals in the country and the hidden dangers inherent in the phenomenon.

7.4 Importance of Bat Coronaviruses

It is an interesting fact that several of the recent pandemics, including SARS, MERS, Ebola, Marburg, and possibly the current novel coronavirus find their origin in bat viruses. Studies concur on the finding that bats' strong immunity pushes viruses to replicate faster, making them ideal hosts for rapidly mutating, and therefore, more deadly viruses. Once these viruses transfer to other mammals, including humans, they wreak havoc on the unsuspecting victims and lead to global contagions. Such conditions make bats unique reservoirs when it comes to rapidly reproducing and highly infectious viruses. Studies also indicate an alarming fact – disruption of bat habitats makes the animals stressed, prompting them to shed more virus through their saliva, faeces and urine, thus potentially causing even greater damage to future hosts.

Even as the pandemic has led to a loss of scores of lives and affected the growth and economic welfare of global countries, studies maintain that bat coronaviruses serve an important purpose. One of the major reasons for this belief is that these viruses draw and enforce the distinction between the human and animal ecosystem, pushing humans to stop encroaching on animal ecosystems. Bats are an important part of nature, they pollinate over 500 plant families and consume harmful mosquitoes, but the consumption of bats, or close contact with the mammals, can lead to zoonotic viral jumps and subsequent pandemic such as the one the world is currently grappling with.

Studies also suggest that bat coronaviruses enforce the law of nature which could be deciphered as a way of prompting humans from resisting when it comes to meat eating, especially in the case of freshly slaughtered and comparatively undercooked or raw meat. Several studies have indicated that the human body functions better on a plant-based diet, as against a meat-based one, and the bat coronaviruses prompt human beings to reconsider and reiterate this theory. Indeed, with the steady stream of scientific research pointing at China's role in the origin of various life-threatening viruses, it is no contest that China's food habits are of concern to the population on a global scale. And, the bat is only one of the dangers when it comes to future pandemics originating in the country.

Chapter 8

"Bat Coronaviruses: The Role of the Furin Cleavage Site"

After a careful study of Animal Viruses over the last 100 years, I have reconfirmed backed by scientific evidence that Bat Coronaviruses (as shown below) have caused the Hendra Virus (Horses), Nipah Virus (Pigs), MERS (Camels), SARS (Civets) & now COVID 19 (Pangolin/Badgers) at various points of time over the last 50-60 years. Please refer to "Clash of 2 Ecosystems", Times of India, Aug 2 & my recent Book, "The Killer Bat", Ashish Kalra, 2021). These Viruses are then transmitted to Humans, when Humans consume these Bat infected Animals. Examples of this are the Asian Flu Pandemic (1957-58),caused by Human Consumption of Ducks (Source: CDC) when over 1.1 million people were killed as also with the SARS Virus (Human consumption of Civets) in 2002 which originated in Guangdong, China and spread to over 32 Countries in less than a month. Same with the MERS Virus (Human Consumption of Camels; Source: WHO), which originated in Saudi Arabia and 27 Countries reported cases. Here also the Virus originated in Bats, and spread to Camels. The intensity of the Viruses has been increasing. MERS was isolated to some degree in the Middle East, hence did not spread. COVID 19 spread because of Chinese tourists post the New Year on 6-7 daily flights to the United States, Europe and Iran. Virus spreads by Aersol Transmission.

    a. **"The Furin Cleavage Site"**: At the heart of these Bat Coronaviruses is a "Furin Cleavage site" which is present in all Coronaviruses (Wao, Zhang: Stem Cell Medicine,2020), which activates a protease enzyme called "furin" which hijacks a protein in our cells. This Furin Cleavage site takes various forms in different

Animals, **but are caused by Bat Coronaviruses.** This is a very important finding.

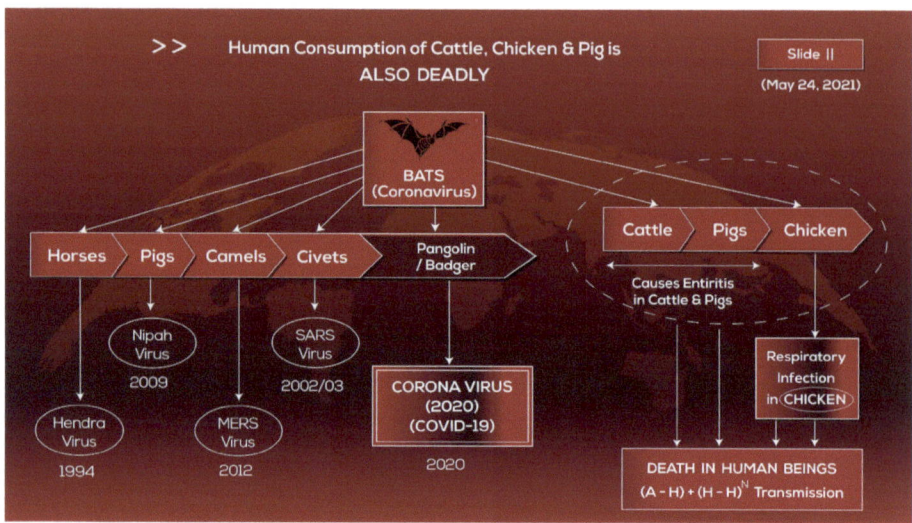

For example, in COVID 19, it has a RBD that binds with high affinity to the Human ACE2 receptor, that hijacks the protein in our cells. The Furin Cleavage site is key in "amplification of the virus" or critical in accelerating its pathogenesis. SARS-COV2 has a polybasic insertion (PRRAR) at the S1/S2 cleavage site that can be "cleaved by furin". Similar action as far as the Furin Cleavage Site in the SARS Virus(Civets). SARS was the Deadly Virus that originated in Guangdong, China in 2002. Sequence alignment of the S1/S2 region in SARS-COV, MERS-COV, SARS-COV2 and Bat Viruses SARSr-COV RaTG13 are closely related to SARS-COV2 (Nature, 579, 270-273, Zhou). This Furin Cleavage site acts when Humans eat these respective Animals-Pangolin/Badgers(COVID 19); Civets (SARS Virus) & MERS Virus(Camels). This hijacks the protein in Human Cells, multiplies and ultimately causes death in Human Beings. Similarly, an analogous "cleavage motif" was present at the S1/S2 of the Spike protein for MERS(Camels) (Scientific Reports 16597, Weber). This spike protein enables MERS(Camels) like Coronaviruses from Bats to infect Human cells. Same as in the case of the Nipah Virus and the role of the "furin cleavage site". A multi-cleavage peptide in the "Nipah Virus" F Protein

(Bat infected Pigs) impairs protolytic processing (Diedrich,PMID 19665506). Similar for the Hendra Virus (Horses). These Furin Cleavage sites are designed to "amplify" these respective "lethal" viruses in Humans; when Humans consume these Animals.

    b. **Human Beings & Animals are Different Ecosystems**: Importantly, these Bat Coronaviruses are structured so that Human Beings cannot encroach on the Animal Ecosystem. Further and importantly, these Bat Coronaviruses also spread to Domestically reared Animals like Cattle, Pigs and Chicken (Perlman & Fehr) causing "fatal" diseases like Entiritis in Cattle & Pigs, Respiratory diseases in Chicken, which get transferred to Humans on consumption & eventually leads to Death in Human Beings. Recently, over 7mn Chickens were culled in Europe recently (potential spread of H5N8 virus from Chickens to Humans). Further, 800,000 Chickens were slaughtered in Russia because of the H5N8 Virus. China reported the H10N3 virus; spread of virus again to Humans. Even when the Chicken is cooked, the virus gets transferred to Humans. Gorman of the New York Times describes this aptly in "A New Bird Flu jumps to Humans"(April 21). In a nut shell, Humans are not designed to eat Animals. Furthermore, Animals are able to absorb these Bat Coronaviruses. Humans cannot. Simply put, Humans cannot encroach on the Animal Ecosystem

    Second, In "Clash of 2 Ecosystems" (Times of India, Kalra, Aug 2). I illustrate the mechanics of [(Animal-Human) + (Human-Human) raise to N transmission] with illustrations from The Asian Flu Pandemic (Ducks, 1958), SARS (Civets, 2002); MERS (Camels, 2012) and now COVID 19 (Pangolin/Badgers). In COVID 19, post the Chinese New Year, passengers from Wuhan travelled to Europe, USA and Iran, spreading the Virus "Human Mouth to Mouth using Aersosol Transmission" ("Optimality of the Virus). The dynamics of COVID 19 are very similar to SARS.

    c. **"Why Plant Based Diets are Critical?"** Third, importantly, Reputed Cleveland Clinic Cardiologist, Dr. Esselstyn's world class research on the criticality of a Plant Based Diet in arresting all forms of "Coronary Disease" (pls read "Preventing and Reversing Heart Disease"). There is a science behind it. Plant based Diet induce the Endothelial Cells to produce Nitric Oxide (1998 Nobel prize awarded to Furchgott, Murad) which is critical in preventing Cardiovascular Disease. This is KEY among other things. This is the Design of Life. The Human Body is Designed to be Vegetarian. Also frequent citations of cases of Colorectal Cancer as a result of "Red Meat consumption" are reinforcements of this argument.

d. **"Design of Human Beings is Vegetarian":** Finally, what we have to bear in mind is that Human Beings are designed to be "Vegetarian", and not Carnivores. Human Beings do not have Canine teeth like Carnivores to tear flesh, have much smaller kidneys than Carnivores, who have have larger kidneys to flush out poisonous meat. Human Beings have much larger intestines like Herbivores, unlike Carnivores which have much smaller intestines. Lastly, Herbivores including Human Beings have much lower levels of hydrochloric acid; Carnivores have high levels of hydrochloric acid to digest meat. Net net, The Design of Human Beings is "Vegetarian", and is similar to Herbivores. To conclude, the "Furin cleavage site" facilitated by Bat Coronaviruses ensures and protects Animals from Human Consumption. Human Beings "cannot encroach" on the Animal Ecosystem. Period. They are different Ecosystems. Similarly, when Cannibals eat Human Beings, they get Brain Disease. The Panacea to get out of this Pandemic and to prevent Future Pandemics is to "Disrupt the Animal Food Chain". Adopt a Plant Based Diet and Lab Based Meat (3 year migration path). Period. Islands like Samoa & Salomon Islands which follow mainly Vegetarian Diets are an important reinforcement point in leadership of a Zero Covid regime. A Tipping Point is when a "series of negative actions act together". Pandemic 2020 is this Tipping Point. "Disrupt the Animal Food Chain". Period.

"Tell me what you eat, and I will tell you what you are"

– **Anthelme Savarin**

Chapter 9

COVID 19: Why Variants Will Defeat Vaccines

The novel coronavirus made its entry towards the end of 2019 and wreaked havoc across the globe in a few months. With scores of infections and multiple deaths, countries began locking their borders and prompting people to remain inside. Social distancing and nationwide lockdowns were mandated in an attempt to control the spread of the virus which did not give in to existing vaccines or known treatment methods. People were scared and panicking, organisations were transitioning to the digital platform, and social life took a nosedive and plummeted to non-existent levels. Even minuscule gatherings for weddings and other social occasions were limited and even there, most people fell prey to the dreaded virus.

The first wave went without offering any ray of hope and the second wave, which began amidst nationwide vaccination drives, claimed an unprecedented number of lives across developing and underdeveloped countries. The virus became a killer that did not spare anyone – people belonging to all categories and demographics fell prey to its infectious nature and rapid transmission. The vaccine, considered the holy grail by many, was developed at a record pace, with countries and premiere research institutions coming up with their own vaccine formulas and standards. People began discussing the merits and demerits of the different formulations and lined up to receive the supposedly life-saving shot.

Even as vaccines were distributed on a national level, news began circulating about an upcoming variant, named the Delta, and research suggested that several vaccines would not be effective in protecting against this variant. The Delta is only one of a number of variants which have cropped up since the novel coronavirus made itself known on a global scale. Which are the other variants which have created panic among the wary populace?

8.1 Various Avatars of COVID

The world has been privy to a number of genetic variants of SARS-CoV-2 since the beginning of the pandemic. These have originated in different parts of the world and circulated through rapid human to human transmission, creating newer varieties of infection and unprecedented number of symptoms. Such mutations are being monitored through sequence-based surveillance, laboratory studies, as well as epidemiological investigations and the only thing conclusive is the fact that the virus is rapidly mutating and taking forms people can only imagine about. According to the Us government's SARS-CoV-2 Interagency Group, there is a variant classification system which enables people to remain aware about the different variants coming up across the globe. The differentiates the variants into three classes – variants of interest, variants of concern, and variants of high consequence.

Under this categorisation, the commonly circulating variants, namely the Alpha, Beta, Delta and Gamma, have been classified as variants of concern. The group is yet to classify a variant as a variant of high consequence, which is a significant relief to the world population. The variants can be differentiated in terms of certain substitutions or combinations of substitutions in their spike protein. Other variants under study include Iota, Kappa, and Eta, and each of their variants have some distinguishing features when it compares with the other virus strains in the coronavirus family. A few of these are of declining prevalence and not of concern and hence, their names are less heard of. At present, it is the new Delta variant which is causing the greatest concern among people.

8.2 Types of Variants

The classification of the different variants depends on how easily they spread, how severe their symptoms are, and how they are treated. A few of the variants are known for rapid infectiousness and this puts a strain on the healthcare system as a larger number of people are infected during the same period of time. This leads to a shortage of healthcare facilities and forces medical professionals to stretch themselves thin while taking care of the patients. Some variants are known to cause severe infection and be unresponsive to treatment, leading to more deaths and all-round suffering. Even in fully-vaccinated individuals, infections are known to take hold and cause complications, though not on as massive a scale as non-vaccinated people. In some variants, there is a possibility of monoclonal treatment not being of great effect.

The surprising number of variants led people to wonder about how many variants are actually extant in the world. Only one thing can be stated as certain – viruses keep altering and this inherent quality and capacity of the virus, to mutate, and transform genetically, leads to the origin of new variants and viral infections. In fact, while people only became aware of the coronavirus family in recent times, following the unprecedented pandemic, it is scientifically proven that the coronavirus has been in existence for a long time. These variants cause a number of illnesses, from mild ones like cough and cold, to serious infections leading to acute respiratory distress and even death. Even the novel coronavirus has existed in the animal ecosystem for a long time, before it jumped into the human body. Therefore, the variant isn't new to the world, it has just made itself known to humans in the recent past.

While the world is now grappling with a number of distinguished virus variants, in early 2020, these many variants had not originated. However, even then, it was clear that there was more than one strain of coronavirus, and these were known to infect different geographical regions and cause different types of symptoms. This quality of the virus also made it difficult for people and medical practitioners to detect the disease conclusively. Treatment was also delayed because of the same. Before the main four virus variants, scientists stated that the coronavirus found in human beings were not all the same. They were distinguished as the "L" and the "S" type, and it is believed that the S type came first. However, the L type is considered more common, especially in the initial phase of the pandemic.

Even as people are getting vaccinated in large numbers, studies state that the virus which causes COVID-19 will most likely keep changing and causing newer infections and symptoms. Further, with the difficulty in predicting how these viruses might change, it becomes even tougher to design vaccines which would be effective against all future variants.

8.3 Causes of the Variants

It is now well known that the coronavirus family consists of a number of fast mutating and dangerous viruses. What is the cause behind this occurrence? What prompts a virus to transition into a new avatar? These are questions which have been doing the rounds since the first variant was discovered and intense research has gone into this query. Research has stated that the more opportunities a virus has to spread, the more it replicates and, with every subsequent replication, its chances of mutating and altering grow tremendously. Therefore, if a virus is widely circulating in a population and triggering multiple infections, as happens during each COVID wave, the possibility of the virus mutating and transforming increases greatly. Studies into the virus' mutations indicate that there is little or no impact on the virus' capability to infect humans or cause symptomatic diseases. However, studies into the virus' genome code indicate that, depending on where the alterations are located on the genetic backbone, the changes may affect properties like transmission and severity. And this has been seen through the study of multiple coronavirus variants, since the beginning of the pandemic.

So how do these variants occur? The coronavirus family has its genetic material in the ribonucleic acid and it is through copying of this RNA that they spread in host cells. Variations in such copying lead to the creation of new strains of virus. These changes are also termed as mutations. In India, the Delta virus was located in October 2020 and was known to be highly contagious. It is causing more cases in young people and has become a dominant strain due to community spread. It is worrisome as the strain is only somewhat responsive to the current vaccines, and that too only after the second dose. In fact, the Delta variant is known to be up to 555 more transmissible when compared to other prevalent strains.

It is also important to note that, with time and vaccination, the new variants are getting stronger and becoming more communicable. Indeed, the more opportunity the virus has to spread, the more mutations it undergoes, making it a potent threat to humanity. Even as scientists are trying to create vaccines which are more effective against existing viruses and potential threats, there is no guarantee as to how effective these could be in the long run. Therefore, it is imperative that people do everything possible to stop the spread to prevent further mutations and origin of additional strains.

8.4 Case Study: The Delta Variant

The Indian-origin Delta variant quickly spread to over 98 countries in a few months, becoming responsible for a vast majority of the case on a global scale. Further, with only parts of the population vaccinated, the Delta variant has a rich and potent field to spread across and mutate further. Almost twice as transmissible as the Wuhan strain, Chinese studies indicate that viral loads in Delta infections are about 1000 times higher than the ones found in other variants. It is regarded as the fastest and fittest variant so far, given its rapid transmission and infectious capabilities. However, while it is more infectious, the symptoms linked to Delta are not very different or more severe than other strains. These include fever, headaches, sore throat, and a running nose.

Exhibit 13: The Delta variant

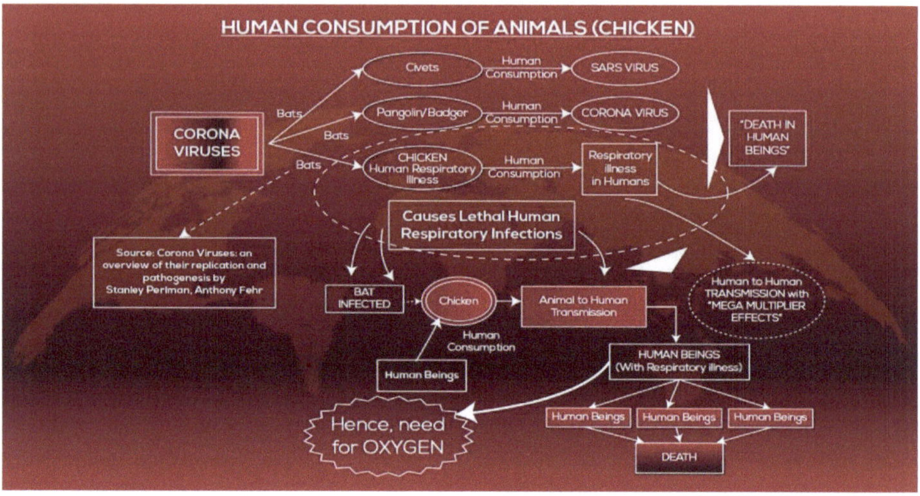

While vaccines are helping reduce mortality and hospitalization in people who have received both doses, neutralization of the Delta variant is not as effective as that of the original strain. In fact, studies state that the Delta strain is 2.9 times less likely to be neutralised with existing vaccines, making people wonder whether variants will defeat vaccines in the long run. A major reason for this concern is the fact that viruses mutate much quicker than the creation of newer vaccines, giving rise to the possibility that variants could, eventually, defeat vaccines.

Multiple case studies indicate that the origin of many variants can be attributed to meat consumption and live produce markets as these create more possibilities of zoonotic transfer and further transmissions between humans. Some researchers have stated that the Delta variant has emerged from the consumption of chicken as this leads to animal-human transmission and chicken have been known to harbour coronavirus strains and fall prey to upper respiratory illness following infections. Following the zoonotic jump from chicken to humans, the virus then transmits from humans to humans, undergoing multiple mutations and genetic alterations along the way. Such mutations then lead to a new variant, which would be additionally unresponsive to existing vaccine formulations.

Further, with India being a country that consumes more of chicken than other animals like pork or beef, there is a higher possibility that the chicken is the source of the new variant. Also, it is fair to state that the Wuhan strain cannot mutate across multiple geographies, leading to the theory that the virus mutations occur within specific geographies, through contact with indigenous animal species who play hosts to the new variants and cause infections in humans. While health organizations across the globe stress on the imperative nature of vaccines, it is no fiction that these vaccines are not completely effective against the new viral strains. In fact, they only offer part efficacy even against the older variants.

Exhibit 14: The need for Oxygen

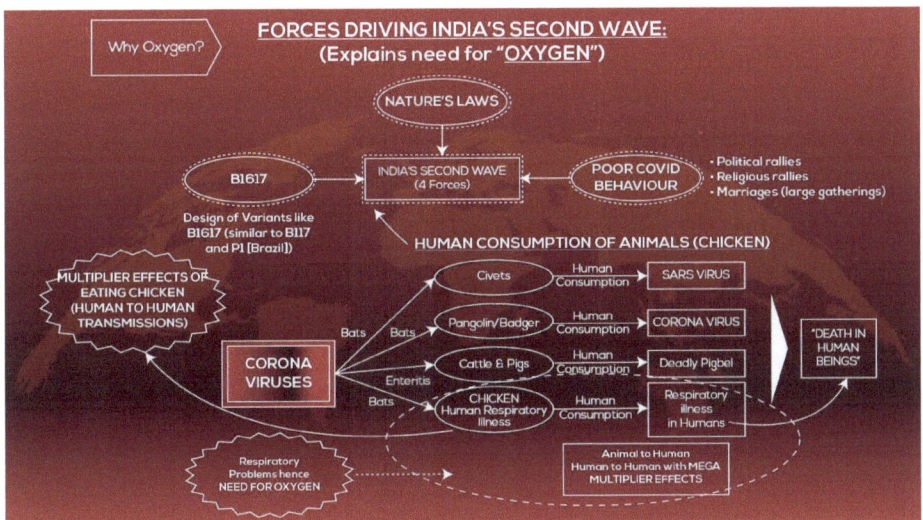

Case studies such as Singapore Airport, Seychelles, and others also show that, despite mass vaccination, people can still fall prey to the newer strains and undergo major illnesses. In such a situation, it leads humans to consider whether it is wise to remain so closely linked with the animal ecosystem, which is the source of most viruses. With the vaccines proving somewhat ineffective against new strains, it is better to maintain a safe distance from potential animal carriers and keep the humankind safe from future virus strains arising out of subsequent zoonotic jumps.

"To become different from what we are, we must have some awareness of what we are"

– **Eric Hoffer**

"This Nitric Oxide Chemistry explains what is perhaps the key mechanism through which my patients became heart attack proof beyond twenty years. "Their Plant based diet" reduced or entirely eliminated all the above cardiovascular risk factors. The more compliant the patient, the more he or she reduced the risks."

– Dr. Caldwell Esselstyn, "Preventing Heart Disease" (Page 43)

Chapter 10

Eleven Madison Park Goes MEATLESS

The COVID-19 pandemic has, in several ways, emphasized on the need for people to go meatless and adopt a more sustainable way of life. It has been proved, time and again, that a variety of the zoonotic viruses, which have wreaked havoc on human beings, have originated in or transferred to people through the close proximity and consumption of animals. And this points to the fact that the animal and human ecosystems are meant to survive co-dependently, one ecosystem is not meant to dominate or diminish the other. In the event of one party attacking the other, the other ecosystem will, in turn, create difficulties for the attacker, leading to death and destruction.

There is Animal to Human Transmission taking place. Now, it does not stop there. There is Human to Human Transmission, sometimes raised to N. This means that not only the person who is Non-Vegetarian is affected, but others as well are affected and killed. For eg in the Asian Flu Pandemic over 2 million perished. Over 4mn Human Beings have perished in COVID 19.

9.1 Biological links between Red Meat and "Colorectal Cancer"

This is one of the other reasons for not eating Red Meat. I draw upon research from Issam Ahmed's work published in Medical Express, June 19'21, "Researchers find biological links between Red Meat and Colorectal Cancer. From the above article, a new paper in Journal "Cancer Discovery" has - now identified specific patterns of DNA damage triggered by diets rich in red meat further implicating the food as a carcinogen while heralding the possibility of detecting the cancer early & designing new treatments. Dana Farber Institute Oncologist, Marias Giannakis who led the study sequenced DNA data from 900 patients with colorectal cancer who were drawn from a much larger group of 28,000 Health workers participating in year long studies. "The analysis revealed a distinct mutational signature- a pattern that had never been before identified but was indicative of DNA damage called "alkylation". Dr. Giannakis explains "With red meat, there are chemicals that cause alkylation". Patients whose tumors had the highest levels of "alkylation damage" had a 47% greater risk of colorectal cancer specific death compared to patients with lower levels of damage.

9.2 President Clinton's "Life Saving Vegan Diet"

One of the inspirations of my research has been the observation of a President Clinton Video on his overcoming Heart Disease, losing weight and leading a Healthier Life using a "Plant based Diet". He cites learnings from eminent Cleveland Clinic Cardiologist, Dr. Caldwell Esselstyn (Cleveland Clinic) and eminent Harvard Medical School Physician, Dr. Dean Ornish.

9.3 "Preventing Heart Disease": The Fantastic Dr. Caldwell Esselstyn Jr

In a fabulous book, "Preventing and Reversing Heart Disease", Dr. Esselstyn outlines the tremendous advantages of adoption of a "Plant Based Diet". He highlights that "Plant based nutrition" has a HUGE BENEFICIAL IMPACT on Endothelial cells (metabolic dynamos) that produce Nitric Oxide. "Nitric Oxide is ABSOLUTELY ESSENTIAL TO Vascular Health". The essential building block for Nitric Oxide Production is a substance called L-arginine, an amino acid that is rich in a variety of plant foods(legumes, beans & nuts (Pg 41,42).

Exhibit 15: Creation of Nitric Oxide is key

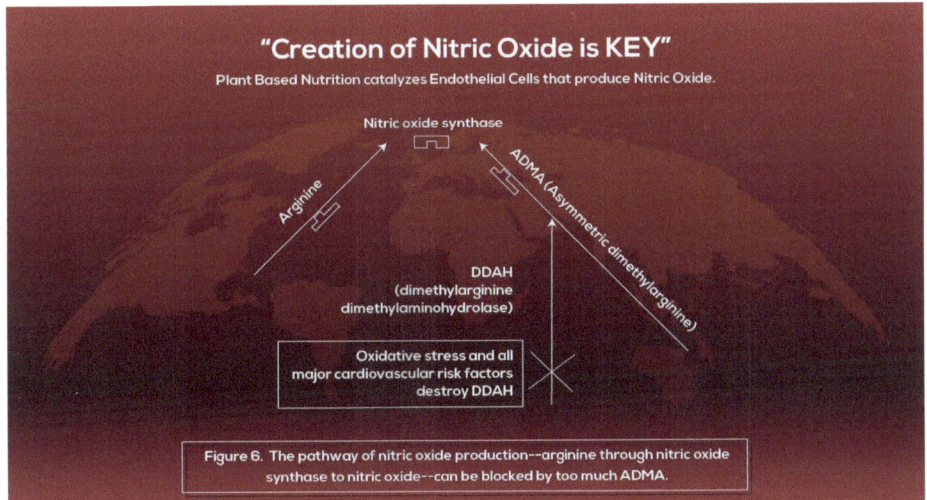

"This Nitric Oxide Chemistry explains what is perhaps the key mechanism through which my patients became heart attack proof beyond twenty years. "Their Plant based diet" reduced or entirely eliminated all the above cardiovascular risk factors. The more compliant the patient, the more he or she reduced the risks."

– Dr. Caldwell Esselstyn, "Preventing Heart Disease" (Page 43)

Symptoms of Acute Respiratory problems being suffered as a result of COVID 19 (SARS- COV2) are identical to those as in SARS-COV (2002, Guangdong, Human Consumption of Bat infected Civets) and during MERS-COV (2012, Middle East, Human Consumption of Bat infected Camel). The exact same symptoms. As shown, Fatigue and Enceliphitis (Swelling of the Human Brain) takes place on consumption of Pigs (CDC). Also, Humans get Abdominal Pain, Chest Pain & Diarrhoea on Consumption of Chicken.

Exhibit 16: The Design of Life

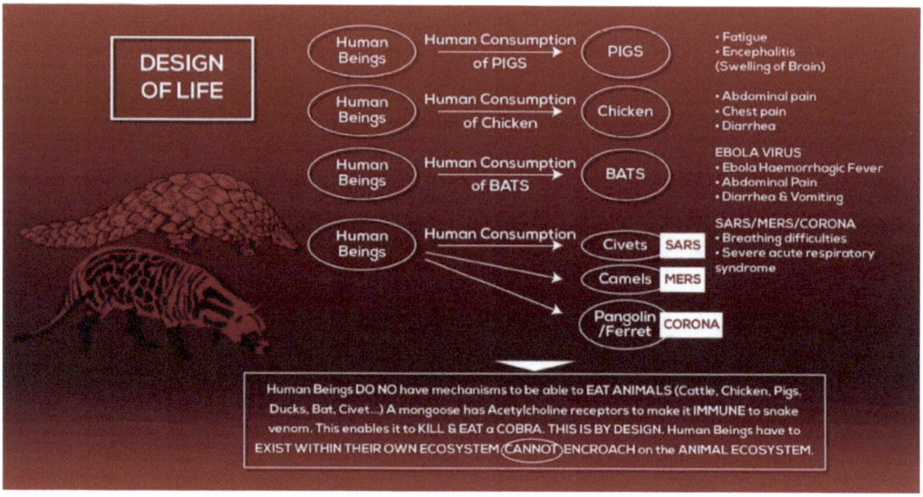

[Diagram: DESIGN OF LIFE]

- Human Beings → Human Consumption of PIGS → PIGS
  - Fatigue
  - Encephalitis (Swelling of Brain)
- Human Beings → Human Consumption of Chicken → Chicken
  - Abdominal pain
  - Chest pain
  - Diarrhea
- Human Beings → Human Consumption of BATS → BATS
  - EBOLA VIRUS
  - Ebola Haemorrhagic Fever
  - Abdominal Pain
  - Diarrhea & Vomiting
- Human Beings → Human Consumption → Civets [SARS], Camels [MERS], Pangolin/Ferret [CORONA]
  - SARS/MERS/CORONA
  - Breathing difficulties
  - Severe acute respiratory syndrome

Human Beings DO NO have mechanisms to be able to EAT ANIMALS (Cattle, Chicken, Pigs, Ducks, Bat, Civet...) A mongoose has Acetylcholine receptors to make it IMMUNE to snake venom. This enables it to KILL & EAT a COBRA. THIS IS BY DESIGN. Human Beings have to EXIST WITHIN THEIR OWN ECOSYSTEM. CANNOT ENCROACH on the ANIMAL ECOSYSTEM.

9.4 Design of 'HUMAN BEINGS IS VEGETARIAN":

Above all, as mentioned in "When we Disobey the Design of Life (Times of India, the Design of Human Beings is "Vegetarian". That is Carnivores have sharp teeth to tear flesh- Herbivores and Man do not. Carnivores gulp down water as against using their mouth and lips (Herbivores). Carnivores have much larger kidneys to flush out poisonous meat compared to Human Beings and Herbivores. Net net, the Design of Human Beings is "Vegetarian".

Exhibit 17: "Plant based Diet is critical"

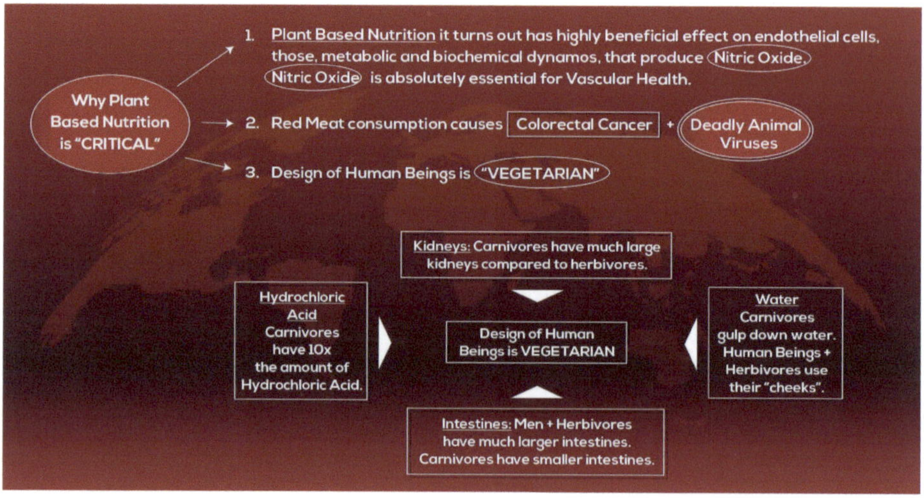

[Diagram: Why Plant Based Nutrition is "CRITICAL"]

1. Plant Based Nutrition it turns out has highly beneficial effect on endothelial cells, those, metabolic and biochemical dynamos, that produce Nitric Oxide. Nitric Oxide is absolutely essential for Vascular Health.
2. Red Meat consumption causes Colorectal Cancer + Deadly Animal Viruses
3. Design of Human Beings is "VEGETARIAN"

Design of Human Beings is VEGETARIAN

- **Kidneys:** Carnivores have much large kidneys compared to herbivores.
- **Hydrochloric Acid:** Carnivores have 10x the amount of Hydrochloric Acid.
- **Water:** Carnivores gulp down water. Human Beings + Herbivores use their "cheeks".
- **Intestines:** Men + Herbivores have much larger intestines. Carnivores have smaller intestines.

One of the recent instances of human beings realizing this phenomenon and taking efforts to relinquish claim on the animal ecosystem is Eleven Madison Park. Several news reports have claimed that the new menu at Eleven Madison Park, front-lined by star chef Daniel Humm, will be meatless. The experienced chef believes that the current food system and diet styles are not sustainable in several different ways. While Eleven Madison Park was previously known for its imported caviar and braised celery root in pigs' bladders, the new menu will completely do away with non-vegetarian cuisines. News reports were rife with the contrast – Eleven Madison Park had gained technical proficiency in creating dishes based on suckling pig, lavender glazed duck and sea urchins, and now, with a focus on sustainability, the restaurant was set to feature a plant-based diet.

9.5 The Eleven Madison Park Story

The volte-face by Eleven Madison Park depicts the upcoming way of life. With more and more people realizing the danger of consuming meat, it is likely that many more individuals will go the Eleven Madison Park route, choosing to relieve their meals of meat and turn to plant-based substitutes which are undoubtedly healthier and significantly less dangerous to human survival. In the words of Ruth Reichel, the reputed editor of the Gourmet Magazine, and a celebrated critic of New York Times, Eleven Madison Park will now function as a teaching institution for people and the impact it will have will be no less than the one exhibited by California's pioneering restaurant – Chez Panisse.

In the original news article in The New York Times, by Brett Anderson and Jenny Gross, the reporters state that Eleven Madison Park is a New York Times four-starred restaurant and also has three Michelin stars, making it a crowd favourite and frontrunner in the food business. With the transformation undertaken by Eleven Madison Park, there is no doubt that fine dine restaurants are keen on revamping and recalibrating themselves in the new normal. Truly, it is not just companies and educational institutes adopting the hybrid way of life, the food business is also set to transform in the new normal. And, with a master chef like Humm leading the way, there is no doubt that more chefs will follow suit in the coming days. And with a refreshing vegetarian palette on offer, it is certain that many non-vegetarians will re-evaluate their eating habits and climb aboard the plant-based bandwagon.

And this transition will not be limited to the food ecosystem – with Humm being a major influencer in today's globalised culture, and people regarding him as one of the finest chefs in the world, there is a strong possibility that Humm's change in outlook could inspire a number of individuals and cultures across the world. Reichel further states that the example set by Humm could reverberate significantly and influence the direction of American cuisine going ahead. It can be argued that not just America, but the world at large, will be impacted by Humm's landmark decision, prompting humanity to take a decisive turn towards the life affirming attitude of vegetarianism.

9.6 Why Chef David Humm's Decision is Imperative

The Eleven Madison Park news comes in the aftermath of one of the worst pandemics endured by the human race. The COVID-19 pandemic, which began in December 2019, has emerged as a black swan event which has caused unprecedented loss of life and livelihood. In fact, as of today, the World Health Organisation pegs the total death, owing to the virus, at 4.5 million, while the total confirmed cases, across the globe, stand at 218.2 million. Almost every country has been affected by the vast transmitting and quickly mutating virus, indicating its expertise in attacking the human populace and causing unnecessary deaths.

Studies have proven that the virus entered human bodies due to consumption of bat-infected mammals, either pangolins or badgers. There is scientific proof that the virus did not emerge in a laboratory in Wuhan, as suggested by multiple conspiracy theorists across the world. With multiple scientists offering their support to the mammal-consumption theory, there is little doubt that the virus originated from natural causes, and spread due to the consumption of mammals in China.

Indeed, China's love for meat consumption has been indicated as the cause behind several of the major virus outbreaks in the world, including the SARS outbreaks since 2000. And these are not isolated incidents. Over the last 100 years, mankind has fought a number of major viral outbreaks, all emerging from the unhindered consumption of meat. These illnesses include avian flues, mad cow disease, swine flu, and Ebola virus, Bats have been identified as the intermediaries in both the recent SARS and MERS outbreaks, as well as the ongoing pandemic.

9.7 Zoonotic Diseases of the 21st Century

A study of the recent zoonotic diseases affecting humans indicates a number of worrisome viral outbreaks. These include the Nipah virus, which proliferated in Malaysia in 1998, where pigs were reared in a bat inhabited region. The virus jumped from the bats to the pigs and then, from the pigs to the humans who consumed them. The humans then transmitted the disease among themselves, leading to an epidemic. The spine flu of 2009, which led to around 3 lakh people being hospitalised, was also caused by pigs. In addition, everything from SARS to MERS and other viral outbreaks have also occurred from human consumption of animals, indicating a strong link between the two events.

Indeed, the ongoing COVID pandemic is extremely similar to the SARS outbreak of 2003 in Guangdong province, China. While the 2003 outbreak was because of humans consuming civets, who were infected by bats, the current pandemic is because of consumption of pangolins or badgers. In every such situation, it is human beings' interference in the animal ecosystem which sets off such dangerous aftershocks, leading to the infection and death of countless people across the world. Even more fearsome is the fact that even vaccines are not entirely effective on these viruses. The recent vaccines have shown around 70-80% efficacy against some strains of COVID, but, with the virus mutating efficiently and quickly, it is likely to be a losing battle on the vaccine's end. And it is a horrendous fact that, despite the number of major viral outbreaks being linked substantially to animal consumption, humans have not yet learned their lesson. In this scenario, Humm's decision comes as an inspiring transformation, something which more people should look towards and follow.

9.8 Assessing COVID-Free Zones

There are some parts of the world which have managed to stay free of the dreaded virus during the global pandemic. While these regions are not large urban settlements with high population densities, they are still examples of how the people's diet in these regions might have saved them from the virus. The Laos, Samoa and Solomon Islands have remained COVID free even as the virus wreaked havoc across global populations and one of the major reasons behind this is the fact that their diet is mostly vegetarian. Their diet includes sweet potatoes, corn, taro roots, cassava, rice, and other vegetables and not killing and eating animals is the major reason for their COVID-free equilibrium. There is, therefore, no doubt that all the viral outbreaks, from SARS to MERS and other flus, have their origin in the consumption of animals, mostly bat-infected ones, and it is this interference, on the human part, which is leading to the origin of life-threatening viruses.

While wild animals are a strict no-no, if the human populace is to be protected from such viral outbreaks, there is also strong support for avoiding the meat of domesticated animals. What is the reason behind this? Top virologists hold that coronaviruses also infect domesticated animals, causing a range of illnesses in animals like cows, pigs, and chickens. Consumption of these animals, once infected, can lead to serious viral outbreaks among human beings, which, once transmitted from human-to-human, can result in deadly pandemics. Animals can fall prey to diseases such as enteritis in cows and pigs, and upper respiratory tract and kidney disease in chickens. Further, the movement of these viruses, from domesticated animals to human beings, results in mega-multiplier effects which leads to tragic death tolls which can be avoided by staying away from meat consumption.

9.9 Possible Alternatives to Meat

It is proven that consuming animals can cause a number of diseases in human beings. Even if only a minority of the population consumes meat, there is still a possibility of infection from non-vegetarians to followers of a plant-based diet. This is not to say that meat should be avoided at all costs. Meat can be consumed, as long as it is not harvested from animals which cause diseases. In this situation, people have the option of depending on lab meat, or meat which is scientifically created in laboratories, without the slaughtering of animals. The combination of a plant-based diet and lab meat can keep human beings healthy and safe, and also prevent viral outbreaks and consecutive deaths.

It is scientifically proven that human beings and animals belong to different ecosystems. These should not intermingle in ways which harm either of the ecosystems. It is when human beings consume animal meat that the other ecosystem harms the human population and causes viral outbreaks. This could be an instance of a natural-built mechanism in animals, which helps protect them from human attacks. It is then understood that human beings should not encroach on the animal ecosystem and this should also include consumption of animal meat.

We can also take survival lessons from the incident at Eleven Madison Park, where the celebrated chef has opted to go the vegetarian way. The restaurant has remained closed since March 2020 and, upon reopening, it would remain dedicated to a plant-based menu, a striking departure from its highly popular meat based creations. The decision came from Humm's understanding of the dangers inherent in the consumption of animal meat. With the pandemic giving rise to several studies which point to the unhygienic conditions in which live stock are held around the world, and the consumption of such meat as the reason for avoidable pandemics, the star chef decided to remove meat from the equation for his patrons. Further, with the pandemic exposing the vulnerabilities in global food supply chains, it made sense to depend on healthy, plant-based alternatives to live animals.

Given Humm's popularity in the fine dining ecosystem, as well as his influence in other cultural settings, there is a strong possibility that Humm's decisive move will go a long way towards prompting people to reassess their meat-eating habits and transition to a plant-based diet which is undoubtedly healthier and safer. The news comes in the wake of the fact that the restaurant has been preparing food boxes for the needy, during the pandemic. This, along with the decision to go vegetarian, indicates Humm's humanitarian and sustainable approach to food and human requirements, making him a good example to look up to. Further, Humm's belief, that human beings' opinion of what constitutes luxury needs to change, is also a thought to give weight to. Indeed, there is no question that we cannot return to the pre-COVID normal. The pandemic has changed a lot for every segment and every individual, and people's food habits post the pandemic should reflect this necessary transformation.

Chapter 11

Why We Need Each Other - "A Nudge to Vegetarianism"

COVID-19, the unprecedented pandemic which is still causing untold damage across the world, has made people evaluate their life choices. The prevalence of zoonotic viruses and outbreaks following human consumption of meat, have led people to question the sense in consuming animal meat. There is growing consensus over the fact that human beings and animals inhabit different ecosystems – one cannot and, more importantly, should not encroach upon the other. It is obvious that nature has created a distinction between the ecosystems for a reason. Human beings are meant to live in harmony with animals, instead of attacking and consuming them. When people forget their place and begin destroying nature, nature reciprocates with a virus as dangerous as the virus we are currently grappling with.

As the creator and purveyor of the things existing within it, nature has charted everything with great scrutiny and accuracy. The disruption of these cycles of life can lead to consequences which have a heinous impact on humanity at large, as we have seen during the current and previous pandemics. With over 4 million deaths on a global scale, and the shutdown of economic and social activities, COVID has impacted humankind like no viral outbreak before it, indicating that, now, it is high time we change our lifestyles and eating habits to a more sustainable version. People are reassessing their lifestyle choices and attempting to make informed decisions and changes to overcome the tragic consequences of the virus. It is, indeed, imperative that we change several things to ensure that such a pandemic does not strike again as even the vaccines are not completely effective against viral outbreaks. COVID has truly shown people the impact of tampering with natural ecosystems and it is high time that humankind learnt their lesson and respected the integrity of natural processes and ecosystems.

11.1 Interconnected Ecosystems

Scientific studies have proven the truth behind the interconnected ecosystems in nature. A popular instance is that of reproduction in rats. Nature has designed rats in a way that they multiply from 2 to 1250 over a single year and this is because rats form the meal of a variety of predatory animals and birds such as falcons, eagles, and owls as well as multiple types of snake variants like pythons, cobras and rattlesnakes. Given the number of animals hunting and feeding on rats, nature ensures that the species do not die out by making them reproduce at an astronomical rate. This is how the equilibrium is maintained in the food chain, ensuring that no animals go hungry or become extinct.

In another instance, the mongoose is equipped with acetylcholine receptors which make them immune to snake venom, ensuring that they can kill even a snake sub-species as poisonous as cobras. Keeping the food chain intact, the mongoose finds its match in raccoons, which are then eaten by jackals who may be eaten by bears. This shows that Animals have a Closed Ecosystem, with every animal playing an important part and it is unwise for human beings to tamper with this ecosystem for their selfish purpose of consuming meat. Human beings should not encroach upon animal ecosystems as this could have disastrous results, as visible during the terrible pandemic we are currently facing.

Exhibit 18: Human disrupting the Animal Food Chain

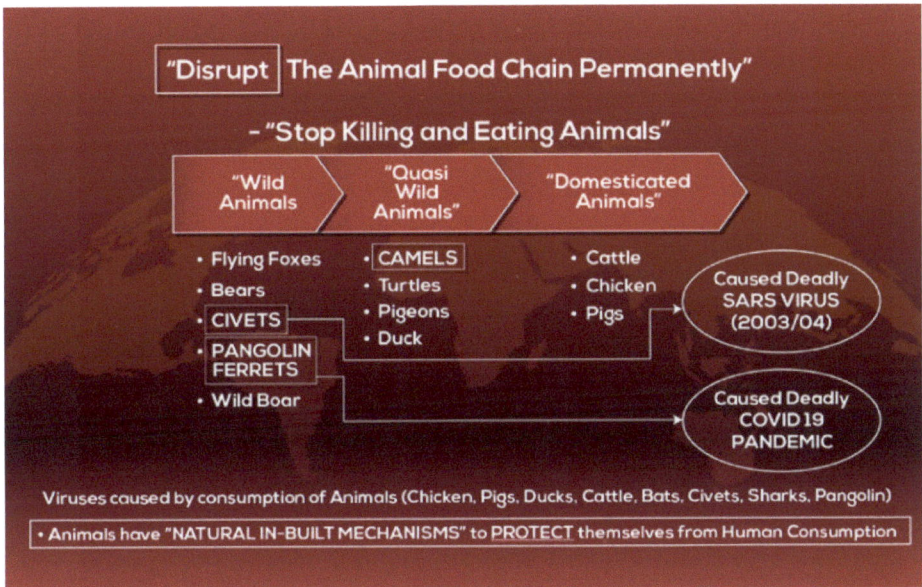

Human beings should stay away from the animal ecosystem as, time and again, it has been indicated that human interference, by way of live produce markets and subsequent consumption of meat, leads to life-threatening diseases such as SARS, MERS, Nipah, swine flu, avian flu, etc. While the coronavirus creates similar symptoms in the bodies it infects, including shortness of breath, severe acute respiratory syndrome and other issues, the vector keeps changing with each virus. While previously SARS was caused by palm civets and camels caused MERS, the ongoing epidemic is likely caused by either pangolins or civets, making it clear that consumption of all animals can disrupt the natural ecosystem and lead to fatal illnesses. It, therefore, can be concluded that human beings have not been designed with the intent of consuming animals and going against this natural design is the cause of most of the recent virus outbreaks. It then stands to reason that, while the virus was not developed in a lab, it is still a man-made virus in the fact that it evolved from human consumption of meat and was, therefore, an avoidable occurrence.

11.2 Maintaining Equilibrium

With humankind facing dire straits due to the virus, which has its origin in meat consumption, it is imperative that mankind reassess its way of life and diet patterns. Additionally, it is also important to control the population, which is rising at an alarming scale, across the world. This is especially necessary in developing countries where people with low incomes go on to have several children, making it difficult to offer proper food and hygienic living conditions. Such scenarios lead to quicker transmission of viruses, making mutations easier and more harmful to human beings. Nations across the globe must work hand in hand to ensure natural equilibrium through promotion of plant-based diets and population control. This is the only way to safeguard humankind from further similar black swan events which could wipe out a majority of the people inhabiting the Earth.

There is no ignoring the network effect indicated by viral outbreaks and consequent deaths. Not only does the infected person end up dying, they also lead to subsequent transmissions and infections which could lead to the deaths of several more people. Nations must, therefore, work towards uplifting each other and helping each other live better and more secure lives. Human beings of any one country cannot survive pandemics without the collaboration of all mankind. Unless every person takes an oath to safeguard the entire human populace, viruses will keep mutating and attacking people, leading to uncountable death tolls and unnecessary loss of lives and livelihoods. Further, while it is understandable that human beings' protein needs may not be met with merely plant-based diets, especially in people who are used to the consumption of animal meat, the transition to laboratory meat is a distinct possibility which offers people all the benefits of meat while also mitigating the possibility of subsequent viral outbreaks caused by human consumption of animals, making it a win-win situation for all involved.

Exhibit 19: The Design of human beings is "Vegetarian":

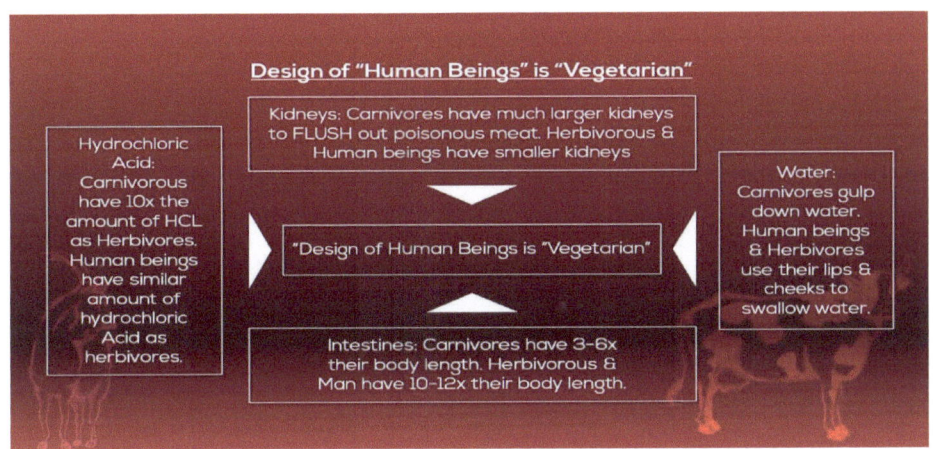

Conclusion

One of the biggest lessons to be learnt from the ongoing COVID-19 pandemic is the fact that, invariably, history repeats itself. We have seen this from the detailed study into how the events during SARS have replicated, on a larger and more infectious scale, during the COVID pandemic we are currently battling. China has been the epicentre of major epidemics, including the SARS infection of 2002-2003. The epidemic created China's greatest socio-political crisis since the 1989 Tiananmen Square massacre and economists believed that the Chinese economy would go into a severe downturn. Everything from the health and security of the Chinese people as well as the entire state of reform, development, and stability were put at risk, along with China's national interest and international image.

Despite the 2002 outbreak, and advancements in the field, China was unable to prevent the outbreak of the ongoing pandemic. Studies suggest that, despite the strong action against SARS in 2002, China's ability to effectively prevent and contain future viruses was uncertain and the blame for this is placed on the fact that prevention and control programmes in the country with the world's largest population are still affected by problems in agenda-setting, policy making, and implementation. Governmental policies and a lack of transparency are considered to be the reasons for this dilemma.

In the present circumstance, vaccines are helping reduce mortality and hospitalization in people who have received both doses but neutralization of the Delta variant is not as effective as that of the original strain. In fact, studies state that the Delta strain is 2.9 times less likely to be neutralised with existing vaccines, making people wonder whether variants will defeat vaccines in the long run. A major reason for this concern is the fact that viruses mutate much quicker than the creation of newer vaccines, giving rise to the possibility that variants could, eventually, defeat vaccines. Case studies such as Singapore Airport, Seychelles, and others also show that, despite mass vaccination, people can still fall prey to the newer strains and undergo major illnesses. In such a situation, it leads humans to consider whether it is wise to remain so closely linked with the animal ecosystem, which is the source of most viruses.

Giving further prominence to the meatless revolution, popular restaurants like Eleven Madison Park are now creating vegetarian menus. It is proven that consuming animals can cause a number of diseases in human beings. Even if only a minority of the population consumes meat, there is still a possibility of infection from non-vegetarians to followers of a plant-based diet. In this situation, people have the option of depending on lab meat, or meat which is scientifically created in laboratories, without the slaughtering of animals. The combination of a plant-based diet and lab meat can keep human beings healthy and safe, and also prevent viral outbreaks and consecutive deaths. We should take survival lessons from the Eleven Madison Park decision, which came from the celebrated chef's understanding of the dangers inherent in the consumption of animal meat.

Another lesson we have learnt is that no nation can survive as a single, insulated unit. With globalisation having made international travel mainstream, people visit different countries frequently and interact with multiple foreigners on a daily basis. In a virus outbreak regime like the one we are currently facing, such travel becomes impossible as it leads to international transmission of viral strains and causes pandemics. With the interconnected nature of human lives, global cooperation is a must when it comes to eradicating or, at least, controlling the impact of the virus and every country on the planet, whether developed, developing or under-developed, must step up to play their part. Collaboration between countries, and symbiotic inter-dependence will help countries move from destructive capitalism to constructive capitalism, indicating a positive equilibrium. Sustainability will be in focus and people will steadily work towards creating a resilient ecosystem capable of living in peace with the animal life cycle.

Additionally, it is not just people or countries that must take efforts to be interdependent. Even ecosystems encompassing global healthcare services should be dependent on each other, especially during such pandemics which put unnecessary pressure on medical supply chains and cause unprecedented loss of health and life. It is imperative that global healthcare systems join hands to ensure the well-being of people across the world as everyone battles the one common enemy – COVID.

The virus has, undoubtedly, caused tremendous loss of life and development and it should be viewed as a lesson for everyone. Human beings cannot, and should not, cross the barriers of animal ecosystems as these lines are created by nature for a specific purpose. It is inadvisable to think that we can continue our lives as they used to be, in the new normal. Indeed, the pandemic is a clarion call for each of us, as individuals and human beings at large, to reassess our lifestyles and eating habits, and arrive at a practice which is both sustainable and in line with the differentiations mandated by nature. Maintaining a healthy lifestyle independent of animal meat consumption is the only way to adapt to the new normal and lead a potentially fulfilling and long life. It is, truly, high time that we learn from the mistakes of our past and create a new lifestyle which is in tune with the ecosystem requirements and adept at mitigating the origin and further evolution of life-threatening human viruses.

www.ingramcontent.com/pod-product-compliance
Lightning Source LLC
Chambersburg PA
CBHW040218220526
45473CB00001B/27